Foreword

As I browsed through the proofs of this excellent book I was reminded that it is just 18 years since, at the request of the Nuffield Provincial Hospitals Trust, I wrote a small monograph entitled *The new genetics and clinical practice*. At that time, recombinant DNA technology was just starting to make its mark on medical research and to demonstrate its likely impact on clinical practice in the immediate future. As I glanced through the chapters of this new book, directed like my monograph at a general medical audience, it was extraordinary to reflect on how much progress had been made over this relatively short period. It is true that, except in the case of clinical genetics, the applications of this new field for day-to-day clinical practice are still limited, but my predictions that in the long term it would have a major impact on medical practice seem to have been vindicated.

It is the very speed of change of the molecular sciences that makes the publication of this book so timely. Bruce Alberts, President of the National Academy of Sciences of the USA, has written recently that the era of molecular biology is already finished. Young biology and medical scientists of the future will have to get to grips with structural biology, biomathematics and information technology. When the Human Genome Project is complete in the early part of the new millennium the central problems of biology will be how to determine the structure and function of proteins from the DNA sequences of their particular genes, and how our hundred thousand or so genes are orchestrated to perform the complex cellular and biochemical interactions that make us what we are. I suspect it will be only when we have this information that the true role of this reductionist approach to human biology and medical research will be fully appreciated.

If research in the new genetics of recent years has told us anything, it is that we are extremely complex animals. Even in the case of the single gene disorders described in this book, where enormous progress has been made towards an understanding of the molecular basis, with a few notable exceptions we have very little idea why the clinical phenotype varies so much from case to case. For the complex multigenic diseases that make up so much of our clinical practice, heart disease, stroke, cancer and the rest, the situation is infinitely more complex. Here, a number of genes are interacting with a wide variety of environmental factors but, as has been so beautifully demonstrated in the cancer field, knowledge of the particular genes involved is likely to tell us a great deal about the underlying cause of these disorders. It also promises to provide the public health field and the pharmaceutical industry with valuable new approaches to their prevention and management. We may even be able to define subsets of our populations at particular high risk for exposure to environmental agents, although I suspect that this type of predictive genetics is, at least in the case of many of our common killers, a long way off in the future.

Like all new advances in medical research and practice, the consequences of the Human Genome Project are raising a number of important ethical issues and problems of regulation, together with genuine difficulties in the public perception of what is going on in the biological sciences. Doctors are one of the major links between science and the community, so it is extremely important that they understand what is happening in this rapidly evolving field and are able to put it into perspective for patients and their families.

We should be grateful to Professors Hughes and Gardiner therefore for drawing together a group of scientists, many of whom are making important contributions to the medical applications of the Human Genome Project, and persuading them to tell us about their work in terms that should be easily accessible to practising clinicians. Even though progress may be less rapid towards the clinical applications of this exciting research than some of the scientists involved have suggested, there is absolutely no doubt that the fruits of the Human Genome Project and the basic biological sciences that relate to it will have an enormous impact right across medical practice in the early part of the new millennium. The true potential of molecular biology for clinical medicine will be realised only if there is continuous and informed communication between practising clinicians and basic scientists. Books of this kind will play an increasingly important role in developing this dialogue; I wish it all the success it deserves.

DAVID J WEATHERALL

September 1998   *Oxford*

Contributors

Eric Alton MD, FRCP *Reader in Thoracic Medicine and Honorary Consultant Physician, Imperial College School of Medicine, National Heart and Lung Institute, Emmanuel Kaye Building, Manresa Road, London SW3 6LR*

Gavin Anderson BSc, MRCP *Wellcome Clinical Training Fellow, Asthma Genetics Group, Nuffield Department of Clinical Medicine, John Radcliffe Hospital, Headington, Oxford OX3 9DU*

Philip Asherson PhD, MRCPsych *Social Genetic and Developmental Psychiatry Research Centre, Institute of Psychiatry, De Crespigny Park, London SE5 8AF*

†**Sarah Bundey** MB, FRCP *Professor of Clinical Genetics, University of Birmingham*

William Cookson MA, DPhil, MD, FRACP *Wellcome Senior Clinical Research Fellow, Asthma Genetics Group, Nuffield Department of Clinical Medicine, John Radcliffe Hospital, Headington, Oxford OX3 9DU*

Sarah Curran PhD, MRCPsych, MRCP *Department of Academic Child Psychiatry, Institute of Psychiatry, De Crespigny Park, London SE5 8AF*

Ian Dunham MA, DPhil *Senior Research Fellow, The Sanger Centre, Wellcome Trust Genome Campus, Hinxton, Cambridge CB10 1SA*

Frances V Elmslie MSc, MRCP *Senior Registrar in Clinical Genetics, Institute of Child Health, Great Ormond Street, London WC1N 3JH*

Rachel Fisher PhD *Cardiovascular Genetics, Department of Medicine, University College London Medical School, The Rayne Institute, University Street, London WC1E 6JJ*

Philippe Froguel MD, PhD *Head of Department – CNRS EP10, Genetics of Multifactorial Diseases, Institut de Biologie de Lille, Institut Pasteur de Lille, 1 rue du Professeur Calmette – BP 245, 59017 Lille Cedex, France*

---

†Sadly deceased.

R Mark Gardiner MD, FRCP *Head, Department of Paediatrics, Royal Free and University College Medical School, University College London, Gower Street Campus, The Rayne Institute, 5 University Street, London WC1E 6JJ*

Andrew J Green MB, PhD, FRCPI *Professor of Medical Genetics, University College Dublin, Faculty of Medicine, and Director, National Centre for Medical Genetics, Our Lady's Hospital for Sick Children, Crumlin, Dublin 12, Ireland*

Peter C Harris PhD, *MRC Senior Scientist, MRC Molecular Haematology Unit, Institute of Molecular Medicine, John Radcliffe Hospital, Headington, Oxford OX3 9DS*

J Ross Hawkins PhD *Lecturer, Molecular Genetics Laboratory, Department of Paediatrics, University of Cambridge, Addenbrooke's Hospital, Box 116, Level 8, Hills Road, Cambridge CB2 2QQ*

Ieuan A Hughes MA, MD, FRCP, FRCP(C), FRCPCH, *Head, Department of Paediatrics, University of Cambridge, Addenbrooke's Hospital, Box 116, Level 8, Hills Road, Cambridge CB2 2QQ*

Steve Humphries PhD, FRCPath, MRCP *Professor of Cardiovascular Genetics, Department of Medicine, University College London Medical School, The Rayne Institute, University Street, London WC1E 6JJ*

Peter Lunt MA, MSc, FRCP *Consultant Clinical Geneticist, Institute of Child Health, Bristol Royal Hospital for Sick Children, St Michael's Hill, Bristol BS2 8BJ*

Chris Mathew *Director, Regional DNA Laboratory South Thames (East), Regional Genetics Centre; and Honorary Senior Lecturer, Guy's Hospital, London Bridge, London SE1 9RT*

George Miller MD, FRCP *Wolfson Institute, St Bartholomew's Hospital, Charterhouse Square, London EC1M 6BQ*

Hugh Montgomery BSc, MB, MRCP *Clinical Lecturer, Hatter Institute for Cardiovascular Studies, Department of Cardiology, University College London Medical School, London WC1E 6JJ*

E Richard Moxon MB, FRCP, FRCPCH *Action Research Professor of Paediatrics, Department of Paediatrics, University of Oxford, John Radcliffe Hospital, Headington, Oxford OX3 9DU*

Marcus E Pembrey BSc, MD, FRCP, FRCOG, FRCPH *Mothercare Professor of Paediatric Genetics, Mothercare Unit of Clinical Genetics and Fetal Medicine, Institute of Child Health, University College London, 30 Guilford Street, London WC1N 1EH*

David Porteous PhD CIBiol, FIBiol *Head, Molecular Genetics Section, MRC Human Genetics Unit, Western General Hospital, Crewe Road, Edinburgh EH4 2XU*

Andrew Read BA, PhD, FRCPath *Professor of Human Genetics, Department of Medical Genetics, St Mary's Hospital, Manchester M13 0JH*

Michele Rees PhD *Senior Lecturer in Molecular Genetics, Department of Paediatrics, Royal Free and University College Medical School, University College London, Gower Street Campus, The Rayne Institute, 5 University Street, London WC1E 6JJ*

Philippa Talmud PhD *Reader in Cardiovascular Genetics, Department of Medicine, University College London Medical School, The Rayne Institute, University Street, London WC1E 6JJ*

Veronica van Heyningen MA, DPhil, MS, FRSE *Section Head, Cell Genetics Section, MRC Human Genetics Unit, Western General Hospital, Crewe Road, Edinburgh EH4 2XU, and Honorary Professor, Faculty of Medicine, University of Edinburgh*

Andrew Wilkie MA, DM, DCH, FRCP *Wellcome Trust Senior Research Fellow in Clinical Science, Institute of Molecular Medicine, John Radcliffe Hospital, Headington, Oxford OX3 9DS, and Honorary Consultant in Clinical Genetics, Department of Medical Genetics, The Churchill, and Oxford Craniofacial Unit, Radcliffe Infirmary*

Tom Wilkie PhD *Head, Biomedical Ethics Section, The Wellcome Trust, 210 Euston Road, London NW1 2BE*

Editors' Introduction

The annual paediatric conference at the Royal College of Physicians, London has given paediatricians over the years a unique opportunity to discuss the pathophysiology of a wide range of disorders of childhood, and to present information about exciting advances in diagnosis and management. In the climate of knowledge which purports to show increasing evidence of a link between the well-being of the fetus and infant and illness in adult life, it is even more important that this conference format is preserved and further developed as a joint activity of the Royal College of Physicians and the Royal College of Paediatrics and Child Health.

When asked by the Academic Board of the Royal College of Paediatrics and Child Health to organise a conference with a genetics theme, we readily accepted the challenge of formulating a programme which would be of interest to a wide range of physicians, be they caring for children or adults. In that context, we decided on the Conference title 'Doctors to the genome'. Perhaps rather speculative, nevertheless no area of medicine is now unaffected by the fruits of the new genetics. Consequently, the conference brief was vast so we were only able to arrange a snapshot of the examples of where medicine (which includes paediatrics) is heading. This book records the edited contributions of the vast majority of conference presentations. The details inevitably become dated, but the principles are accurate, profound and set the scene for the future. We report with much regret that Sarah Bundey, who contributed so much to the understanding of the genetics of mental retardation, died while this book was in preparation.

Once the conference programme had been finalised, the editors had a relatively easy and pleasant task to produce the proceedings. To all the authors and also to the RCP publications department, we express our deep appreciation and gratitude.

IEUAN HUGHES and MARK GARDINER
December 1998

Contents

Part 2. A spectrum of single gene disorders – an update

Part 3. The 1997 Teale Lecture

Part 4. Complex multigene disorders

Part 5. Future prospects

1 | Historical overview of the genetic revolution

Marcus Pembrey
Institute of Child Health, University College London

The genetic revolution may be viewed as having five main components:

- molecular genetic techniques;
- research strategies;
- genetic mechanisms/concepts;
- clinical genetic services; and
- public policy.

The way in which the *molecular techniques* and *research strategies* have fed into clinical diagnostic services is illustrated in Table 1. The molecular pathology of the haemoglobinopathies is used as an example because our understanding of them has usually been ahead of that of most other diseases. By the mid-1980s, most information was in place for mapping disease gene loci using linkage analysis and, with the development of physical mapping tools such as yeast artificial chromosomes, for the positional cloning of mutant genes (eg cystic fibrosis transmembrane regulator gene in 1989).

The three major surprises in terms of *genetic concepts and mechanisms* are the following:

- Genes are split into introns and exons (in 1977).
- Trinucleotide repeat sequences can expand from one generation to the next, for example, dynamic mutations in fragile X syndrome, myotonic dystrophy and Huntington's disease (early 1990s).
- The expression of some genes is dependent on the sex of the transmitting parent: genomic imprinting (late 1980s).

The UK has perhaps fared better than many countries in terms of the development of *public policy* and *clinical genetic services*. The academic centres of medical genetics gave birth to the National Health Service network of regional clinical genetic centres. With

1

Table 1. The chronological development of molecular technologies, research strategies and their introduction into clinical genetic services (1949–85).

	Molecular genetics		Molecular pathology (of haemoglobins)
Year	Event	Year	Event
1953–mid 60s	DNA structure Transcription Translation Genetic code	1949	Sickle haemoglobin shown to be a defect in the structure of globin component
1968–71	DNA sequence-specific restriction	1958	Amino acid substitution shown in sickle haemoglobin (β^s)
1970	Reverse transcriptase	1960s	Abnormal haemoglobins and thalassaemias
1973	Plasmid cloning recombinant DNA in *Escherichia coli*	1976	Prenatal diagnosis using gene-specific probe
1977	Introns and exons of genes	1978	Genetic test exploiting linkage disequilibrium of β^s to an RFLP 1981–82
1980	Linkage map with RFLPs	1981–82	Prenatal DNA diagnosis on chorionic villus biopsy
1985	Polymerase chain reaction		

1985–90
British DoH evaluation of DNA analysis in clinical genetic services
Cardiff, Manchester, London (Institute of Child Health)

DoH = Department of Health
RFLP = restriction fragment length polymorphism

the support of the Royal Colleges, a firm professional framework for clinical genetics was established, leading to specialty recognition in 1980. Importantly, this allowed the benefits of genetic and related research to be demonstrated in terms of patient services when public debate increased. The debate on genetics, in the UK at least, developed largely on the back of the remarkable public discussion in the 1980s about *in vitro* fertilisation, embryo research and pre-implantation genetic diagnosis, culminating in the Human Fertilisation and Embryology Act, 1990. This, in turn, established a professional/public dialogue that effectively informed the House of Commons Science and Technology Committee in 1994–95. Its report *Human genetics: the science and its consequence*[1] led to the establishment of the Human Genetics Advisory Commission (Department of Trade and Industry, and the Department of Health (DoH)), which coincidentally held its first meeting on the day the birth of the cloned sheep, Dolly, was announced! This Commission, the DoH Advisory Committee on Genetic Testing and the Gene Therapy Advisory Committee provide an advisory framework that should enhance the benefits and temper the fears that may come with the genetic revolution.

Reference

1   Third report of the House of Commons Science and Technology Committee. *Human genetics: the science and its consequence*, vol 1. London: HMSO, 1995.

Part 1

The genome project

2 | The mouse and the human genome project

Michele Rees
Department of Paediatrics, The Rayne Institute,
Royal Free and University College Medical School

The mouse as a model organism

The mouse has become the primary model organism for the human genome project, for several cogent reasons. In the literature there are about 600 well documented mutant mouse strains affecting a diversity of biological systems and pathways,[1] many of which share phenotypic similarities with human genetic diseases. In studying such mutations, the mouse has the distinct advantage that it can be crossed in sufficient numbers and with sufficient ease to enable the mapping of both simple (ie single gene) and complex genetic traits.

A major breakthrough in facilitating such studies was the advent of the interspecific backcross,[2] which enables many hundreds of informative recombinant offspring to be rapidly produced. Because of the high density of the current mouse genetic map and the thousands of available polymorphic markers, DNA from these animals can rapidly be typed by means of the polymerase chain reaction, and the map location of the mutated gene determined. A mouse cross of 1,000 animals theoretically enables the location of a particular gene to be determined to within 0.1 cM. In the mouse, on average, this represents a physical distance of only 200 kb. Such a small distance is easily accessible to modern gene isolation techniques.

The mouse genome is therefore much more easily manipulated than the human genome. Mapping of a particular genetic trait in humans is reliant on the availability of good (ideally large) informative families, and the genetic resolution obtained from such mapping studies may be relatively low. In addition, a mouse interspecific backcross has an advantage in that it is genetically homogeneous (ie the same gene is mutated in all affected animals), whereas in humans different families may possess mutations in

7

distinct genes making linkage analysis difficult (although not impossible).

In addition to the availability of a large number of mutant strains, comparative studies are aided by the remarkable similarity of the mouse and human genomes. Despite their evolutionary divergence over 80 million years ago, they are of similar size (ca 3×10^9 bp) and contain comparable repertoires of genes. Comparison of genetic maps of the mouse and human indicates large stretches of chromosomes where both gene content and gene order are conserved (for an example, see Fig 1). These *conserved linkage groups* are well documented and span the majority of the mouse and human genomes (reviewed in Ref 3). This information enables the

Human		Mouse	
Chromosome	**Gene**	**Chromosome**	**Gene**
2p25	ACP1	Acp1	12
2p25-p24	TPO	Tpo	12
2p25-p24	RRM2	Rrm2	12
2p25	ODC1	Odc	12
2p23	POMC	Pomc1	12
2p24.1	MYCN	Nmyc1	12
2p24-P22	ADCY3	Adcy3	12
2p24-p23	APOB	Apob	12
2p	SDC	Synd1	12
2p12	REG1A	Reg1a	12
2p22-21	HSOS1	Sos1	17
2p22-21	PRKR	Prkr	17
2p22-21	MSH2	Msh2	17
2p21	LHCGR	Lhcgr	17
2p22	XDH	Xdh	17
2p21	SPTBN1	Spnb2	11
2p13-p12	REL	Rel	11
2p13	ANX4	Anx4	6
2p13	TGFA	Tgfa	6
2p13	EGR4	Egr4	6
2p13-p12	MAD	Mad	6
2p12-p11.1	CTNNA2	Catna2	6
2p	SFTP3	Sftp3	6
2p12	CD8A	Cd8a	6
2p12	CD8B1	Cd8b	6
2p11	FABP1	Fabp1	6
2p12	IGK	Igk	6

Fig 1. *Comparative gene map of the short arm of human chromosome 2 illustrating the existence of four identified conserved linkage groups on mouse chromosomes 6, 11, 12 and 17* (adapted from Ref 3).

map location of a gene in one species to be used with reasonable accuracy to predict the likely location of its orthologue in the other species.

Table 1 illustrates a few of the recently cloned mouse genes which give rise to particular neurological phenotypes (although, as stated previously, many other mutations affecting other biological systems also exist) in which mutations have been shown to cause homologous disorders in humans. For example, mutations in the peripherin-2 gene, which underlies a proportion of cases of autosomal dominant retinitis pigmentosa, were discovered only following the demonstration of a mutation in the homologous gene in the *retinal degeneration slow* mutant.[4,5] The glycine receptor α1 (*GLRA1*) gene is mutated in the rare autosomal dominant human disorder hyperekplexia (or startle disease) and its murine orthologue *Glra1* is also mutated in the *spasmodic* mouse mutant.[6,7] Studies of several mouse deafness mutants have increased understanding of the underlying causes and mechanisms of human deafness.[8-12] It can be assumed that other, as yet unidentified, mouse mutations will continue to aid the study of human disease.

Mouse models and mechanisms underlying human genetic diseases

The two major ways in which mouse models have contributed to our knowledge of the mechanisms underlying human genetic diseases are discussed below, with some appropriate examples.

Mapping/cloning of the homologous mouse gene

Conserved linkage groups in the mouse and human genomes may enable the map location of a gene in the mouse to be used to predict the likely location of the homologous gene in man. Several human diseases have benefited from mapping studies in the mouse.

The genetics of deafness. One of the best examples of a disease that has benefited is deafness. The complex morphology of the inner ear indicates that a large number of genes are involved in its development and function, and mutations at numerous distinct loci have been found to cause deafness in both humans and mice (for more comprehensive reviews see Refs 13–15). It is estimated that about one in 2,000 children is born with a genetic hearing impairment, about two-thirds of these show an autosomal recessive inheritance

Table 1. Examples of mouse neurological phenotypes and homologous human disorders.

Mouse mutant				Chromosome	
Name	Symbol	Human disorder	Gene product	Mouse	Human
retinal degeneration slow	*rds*	retinitis pigmentosa	peripherin-2	17	6p21-cen
shaker-1	*sh-1*	Usher 1B	myosin VIIA	7	11q13
small eye	*sey*	aniridia	Pax6	2	11p13
spasmodic	*spd*	hyperekplexia	Glycine receptor α1 subunit	11	5q32
splotch	*sp*	Waardenburg type 1	Pax3	2	20p11
tottering	*tg*	FHM	calcium channel	8	19p13
		EA type II	α1 subunit		
		SCA type 6			
	mdx	DMD	dystrophin	X	X

mdx = X-linked muscular dystrophy
DMD = Duchenne muscular dystrophy
EA = episodic ataxia
FHM = familial hemiplegic migraine
SCA = spinocerebellar ataxia

pattern, another one-third display autosomal dominant inheritance, and 1–2% show X-linked inheritance. Some of these cases are syndromic in that they also include other phenotypic characteristics which aid diagnosis. Several genes underlying syndromic deafness have been identified including, for example, *PAX3* mutations in the *splotch* (*sp*) mutant and Waardenburg syndrome type 1,[16] and the *MITF* gene in the mouse *microphthalmia* (*mi*) mutant and in Waardenburg syndrome type 2.[17]

In contrast, non-syndromic deafness has traditionally been much more difficult to study since it is known to be genetically heterogeneous. However, several loci for both autosomal dominant and autosomal recessive non-syndromic deafness have now been mapped. This is an example of a defect in which the identification of the underlying genes may be speeded up considerably by the study of relevant mouse models.

The shaker-1 (sh-1) mouse. The *sh-1* mouse is an autosomal recessive mutation which displays both hearing impairment and vestibular abnormalities due to a neuroepithelial abnormality primarily involving the organ of Corti. The *sh-1* gene was originally mapped to mouse chromosome 7. It was cloned using a large interspecific backcross and found to be an unconventional myosin, myosin VIIA, expressed in the hair cells of the inner ear.[8] The region of chromosome 7 to which this gene was mapped was known to show conservation of linkage with human chromosome 11q13.5. This is a region of the human genome to which, coincidentally, a gene for Usher's syndrome type 1B and for a type of non-syndromic autosomal recessive deafness had been localised. Usher's syndrome is a type of syndromic deafness (DFNB2) in which affected individuals also display retinitis pigmentosa. On examination of the human myosin VIIA gene, mutations were discovered in Usher's syndrome patients.[10] More recently, mutations in the same gene have been shown also to underlie DFNB2.[11,12] The *sh-1* mouse mutant has therefore been instrumental in unravelling aspects of both syndromic and non-syndromic deafness in terms both of the genes and types of mutations involved and of the mechanisms of action of the gene products.

Some of the mapped human autosomal recessive deafness loci, together with their potential murine homologues, are illustrated in Table 2. There are several mapped autosomal dominant non-syndromic deafness loci that may also be shown to possess murine homologues (reviewed in Ref 15). It seems likely, therefore, that at least some of the other numerous mouse deafness mutations

Table 2. Potential human autosomal recessive deafness loci and their murine homologues (adapted from Ref 15).

Locus	Human chromosome	Corresponding mouse chromosome	Candidate mouse mutants
DFNB2	11q13.5	7	shaker-1
DFNB3	17p11.2-q12	11	shaker-2
DFNB4	7q31	6	sightless
DFNB5	14q12	14	
DFNB6	3p14-p21	9	spinner
		14	
		6	
DFNB7	9q13-q21	19	deafness
		13	
DFNB12	10q21-q22	10	Waltzer
			Jackson circler
			Ames waltzer

will have direct human homologues, so the mouse will be a useful tool in dissecting the genetics of deafness for some time to come.

Highlighting a novel mechanism or class of genes possibly involved in complex human genetic diseases

Mapping in the mouse to provide clues as to the map location and identity of the corresponding human gene has been applied mainly to disorders in which the inheritance pattern is Mendelian (ie either dominant or recessive). In many common disorders in humans, however, there is a clear genetic predisposition but the inheritance pattern is unclear. This may be due either to the effects of several genes interacting with each other or to the external effects of the environment influencing genetic predisposition to developing a particular condition. Genes for so-called *quantitative trait loci* can be mapped in the mouse. This has been done for several complex disorders (eg epilepsy), but the relatively low genetic resolution of this approach renders positional cloning of the underlying genes a difficult task.

Single gene defects in the mouse may shed light on a category of genes or on a particular metabolic pathway which may be defective in similar human disorders with a complex inheritance pattern. Examples of the types of disorder in which this approach has been applied include epilepsy, diabetes and obesity. Mouse models of obesity are discussed below.

Mouse models of obesity

Several single gene defects in the mouse result in obesity of varying degrees and age of onset. The most extensively studied is probably the obese (*ob*) mouse, an autosomal recessive defect which results in early-onset profound obesity giving rise to affected mice about twice the weight of their normal litter mates. The *ob* gene was originally mapped to chromosome 6. Positional cloning by Friedman and colleagues[18] identified a novel gene, the product of which was called 'leptin' (from the Greek *leptos* meaning 'thin').

Leptin

Leptin has been shown to be a circulating hormone secreted exclusively by adipose tissue; it acts on the hypothalamus as a satiety factor to control both appetite and energy expenditure. In humans, segregation analyses in different populations indicate that up to 80% of risk for obesity is conferred by genetic factors. Genetic linkage analysis in humans suggests that the human '*ob*' locus plays a role in body fat content (reviewed in Ref 19), but several studies have shown no evidence for mutations which would disrupt the function of the gene.

In June 1997, a paper in *Nature*[20] described a congenital leptin deficiency associated with extremely severe early-onset obesity in humans in a rare consanguineous Asian pedigree with an autosomal recessive mode of inheritance. This was really the first demonstration that leptin plays an integral role in the control of appetite and body fat stores in humans. It remains to be seen whether more subtle variations in the leptin gene are responsible for less severe cases of this common disorder. Additional evidence of the importance of this pathway comes from the observation that the gene underlying another obese mouse mutant, diabetes (*db*) mouse, encodes the hypothalamic receptor for leptin,[21,22] and that this gene is also mutated in the fatty (*fat*) rat model.[23]

Studies of several mouse models of obesity have therefore been the key to discovering a novel pathway controlling appetite and energy expenditure in the mouse which may play an equally important role in humans.

The genes responsible for several additional obesity mutants have also now been cloned (Table 3). Their identification indicates

Table 3. Cloned mouse obesity genes.

Mutant	Symbol	Onset	Gene product
obese	*ob*	very early	leptin
diabetes	*db*	early	leptin receptor
agouti yellow	A^y		ectopic expression of secreted protein
fat	*fat*	maturity	carboxypeptidase E
tubby	*tub*	maturity (3–6 months)	novel hydrophilic protein
fatty zucker*	*fa*		leptin receptor

*rat model

several classes of candidate genes which deserve thorough investigation, but it remains to be seen whether any of these play a significant role in the control of body fat in humans.

Future prospects

There are several ways in which mouse mutants can aid the study of human genetic diseases and also give insights into the processes controlling normal biological functions. In addition to allowing the study of the underlying pathophysiology of such diseases, by enabling easy access to the affected tissues such models also provide an invaluable *in vivo* experimental framework for exploring the efficacy of novel therapies. It must be stressed that there are many mouse mutants for which the genes have yet to be cloned and which may extend the catalogue of murine homologues of human diseases. It seems likely that the mouse will continue to be a valuable aid to the human genome project for the foreseeable future.

References

1 Doolittle D, Davisson MT, Guidi JN, Green MC. Catalog of mutant genes and polymorphic loci. In: Lyon M, Brown S, Rastan S (eds). *Genetic variants and strains of the laboratory mouse.* Oxford: Oxford University Press, 1996: 17–854.
2 Avner P, Amar L, Dandolo L, Guenet JL. Genetic analysis of the mouse using interspecific crosses. *Trends in Genetics* 1988; **4**: 18–23.
3 Meisler M. The role of the laboratory mouse in the human genome project. *American Journal of Human Genetics* 1996; **59**: 764–71.
4 Farrar GJ, Kenna P, Jordan SA, Kumar-Singh R, *et al.* A three-base pair

deletion in the peripherin-RDS gene in one form of retinitis pigmentosa. *Nature* 1991; **354**: 478–80.

5   Kajiwara K, Hahn LB, Mukai S, Travis GH, *et al.* Mutations in the human retinal degeneration slow gene in autosomal dominant retinitis pigmentosa. *Nature* 1991; **354**: 480–2.

6   Kingsmore SF, Giros B, Suh D, Bieniarz M, *et al.* Glycine receptor β-subunit gene mutation in *spastic* mouse associated with LINE-1 element insertion. *Nature Genetics* 1994; **7**: 136–42.

7   Shiang R, Ryan SG, Zhu Y-Z, Hahn AF, *et al.* Mutations in the α1 subunit of the inhibitory glycine receptor cause the dominant neurologic disorder, hyperekplexia. *Nature Genetics* 1993; **5**: 351–8.

8   Gibson F, Walsh J, Mburu P, Varela A, *et al.* A type VII myosin encoded by the mouse deafness gene shaker-1. *Nature* 1995; **374**: 62–4.

9   Avraham KB, Hasson T, Steel KP, Kingsley DM, *et al.* The mouse Snell's waltzer deafness gene encodes an unconventional myosin required for structural integrity of inner ear hair cells. *Nature Genetics* 1995; **11**: 369–75.

10 Weil D, Blanchard S, Kaplan J, Guilford P, *et al.* Defective myosin VIIA gene responsible for Usher syndrome type 1B. *Nature* 1995; **374**: 60–1.

11 Weil D, Kussel P, Blanchard S, Levy G, *et al.* The autosomal recessive isolated deafness, DFNB2, and the Usher 1B syndrome are allelic defects of the myosin-VIIA gene. *Nature Genetics* 1997; **16**: 191–3.

12 Liu X-Z, Walsh J, Mburu P, Kendrick-Jones J, *et al.* Mutations in the myosin VIIA gene cause non-syndromic recessive deafness. *Nature Genetics* 1997; **16**: 188–90.

13 Brown S, Steel K. Genetic deafness – progress with mouse models. *Human Molecular Genetics* 1994; **3**: 1453–6.

14 Steel K, Brown S. Genes and deafness. *Trends in Genetics* 1994; **10**: 428–35.

15 Petit C. Genes responsible for human hereditary deafness: symphony of a thousand. *Nature Genetics* 1996; **14**: 385–91.

16 Tassabehji M, Newton VE, Leverton K, Turnbull K, *et al.* PAX3 gene structure and mutations: close analogies between Waardenburg syndrome and the Splotch mouse. *Human Molecular Genetics* 1994; **3**: 1069–74.

17 Tassabehji M, Newton V, Read A. Waardenburg syndrome type 2 caused by mutations in the human microphthalmia (MITF) gene. *Nature Genetics* 1994; **8**: 209–10.

18 Zhang Y, Proenca R, Maffei M, Baronc M, *et al.* Positional cloning of the mouse obese gene and its human homologue. *Nature* 1994; **372**: 425–32.

19 Leibel RL. And finally, genes for human obesity. *Nature Genetics* 1997; **16**: 218–20.

20 Montague CT, Farooqi IS, Whitehead JP, Soos MA, *et al.* Congenital leptin deficiency is associated with severe early-onset obesity in humans. *Nature* 1997; **387**: 903–8.

21 Chen H, Charlat O, Tartaglia LA, Woolf EA, *et al.* Evidence that the diabetes gene encodes the leptin receptor: identification of a mutation in the leptin receptor gene in db/db mice. *Cell* 1996; **84**: 491–5.

22 Lee G-H, Proenca R, Montez JM, Carroll KM, *et al.* Abnormal splicing of the leptin receptor in diabetic mice. *Nature* 1996; **379**: 632–5.

23 Phillips MS, Liu Q, Hammond HA, Dugan V, *et al.* Leptin receptor missense mutation in the fatty zucker rat. *Nature Genetics* 1996; **13**: 18–9.

3 | The human genome project and genome sequencing

Ian Dunham

The Sanger Centre, Wellcome Trust Genome Campus, Cambridge

This chapter will provide an overview of the human genome project (HGP) and its current status, and also some discussion of genomic sequencing and the question 'why sequence genomes?'. First, at least some of the socio-political background out of which the project has arisen will be described. This will be followed by summarising the progress of the HGP in most of its key areas, indicating how this progress is relevant to medical genetics. Finally, some issues about genomic sequencing, particularly of man, will be addressed.

Socio-political background to the human genome project

A number of prominent molecular biologists have essentially campaigned for the sequence of the human genome to be determined since the late 1980s (eg see Ref 1). Walter Gilbert famously called the human genome sequence the 'grail of human genetics'. Other phrases, such as the 'blueprint of life' and the 'Everest of molecular biology', have been often repeated in the context of the HGP. Francis Collins, current Director of the National Institutes of Health National Human Genome Research Institute, has portrayed the HGP as comparable to putting a man on the moon, or splitting the atom.[2] This hyperbole is motivated by these molecular biologists' belief that the knowledge derived from the human genome will be incredibly powerful for biology and medicine, and that the systematic approach to the human genome will eventually be the most efficient means to approach those human diseases which have a genetic component.

The drive to 'know thyself' in terms of our genomes has also sharpened our perspective on the ethical and philosophical issues involved in the use of genetic information. These issues are dealt with in more detail in other chapters, but must be kept in mind

17

when reviewing the status of the HGP. Certainly in the media and among the general public there is a feeling that the information provided by the HGP will be powerful – but we do not yet know *how* powerful. This uncertainty is expressed well by Philip Kitcher in *The lives to come. The genetic revolution and human possibilities*:[3]

> Alternately inspiring and appalling, kaleidoscopic images of possible futures whirl by. We sense that the molecular revolution will make large differences – how large, we do not know – in the lives our children will lead, we sense that we have the power now to channel the impact the new biology will have on society, but the kaleidoscope moves too quickly. We do not know how to stop it, how to bring these images into focus, how to decide which of them represents something for which we should genuinely hope or of which we have reason to be afraid.

It is against this background that the HGP continues to accelerate, so much so, in fact, that some have confidently predicted that we will have the complete human genome sequence before the middle of the next decade.[4] This chapter reports on what has been achieved thus far.

What is the human genome project?

The motivation behind the HGP is based upon the molecular genetic paradigm, that the biology and medicine of human beings are determined by the interaction of the products of our genetic complement with each other and with the environment. If, therefore, all the building blocks of the genetic human were known, biology and medicine could be approached systematically and genetically. Another way of phrasing this reductionist approach is to say that it would be much easier to solve the human genetic jigsaw if we knew we had all the pieces. The widespread acceptance of this paradigm led to the birth of the HGP, the most concise definition of which is that it is a 15-year global initiative to discover all the human genes. This aim is being achieved through a series of scientific strategies, which include:

- human genetic and physical map making;
- genomic and cDNA sequencing; and
- work on the genomes of model organisms such as the mouse, the nematode *Caenorhabditis elegans*, the yeast *Saccharomyces cerevisiae* and the fruit fly *Drosophila melanogaster*.

The time scale refers specifically to the US HGP which started officially in 1991.[5] The start can, however, be traced back to the mid-1980s, and in this author's opinion, it will continue in various forms beyond 2006 even if the genome is fully sequenced. The project is international: at least 17 countries have a government funded HGP, and the umbrella organisation for human genome investigators, the Human Genome Organisation (HUGO), has over 1,000 members from 50 countries.[6] Although international, it is funded nationally and implemented through many institutions. The necessary coordination is achieved nationally through the funding bodies, and internationally through organisations such as HUGO and international strategy meetings such as those held in Bermuda in 1996 and 1997.[7]

What will the human genome project deliver?

If the aim of the HGP stated above is achieved, all the human genes will have been discovered. In practice, this will be achieved through a series of technologies and strategies, each of which can provide quantifiable products. For the clinical geneticist, the motivation must be to know all the genes involved in human genetic disease. Several of the products of the HGP are immediately available to aid this:

- The genetic or meiotic map allows the localisation of a gene for a particular disease to a region of the genome.
- The physical map allows direct access to the DNA at that location.
- The transcript map places a series of candidate genes into the genetic locality.
- The human genome DNA sequence places all genetic information on a common information infrastructure (an encyclopaedia of human genes) which is available for study in medicine and biology.

The human genome project product

The HGP product will contain all the genes and allow the researcher to go direct from genetic mapping to the complete set of testable candidate genes for a disease. It is important to point out that the HGP product will necessarily be a composite, a mosaic, of several human genomes. Except for identical twins, it is estimated that any two human genomes will differ from each other at three million positions. There is not one bench-mark human genome or sequence, but a population of different genomes. The methodology of the HGP will produce a composite of these, but the HGP product will allow the differences between genomes to be investigated. It is this variation in the genetic complement and its interaction with the environment that are responsible both for the differences between people and for what we call 'disease'.

The scale of the problem and the solution

The human genome comprises 3,000,000,000 bp of DNA (3,000 Mb) packaged into 22 pairs of autosomes, plus the two sex chromosomes, X and Y, and is estimated to contain upwards of 60,000 genes.[8] However, perhaps 30% of the DNA is comprised of tandem and dispersed repetitive DNA elements (eg α satellite, *Alu* repeats). The genes can vary in size from a few kb to 2 Mb. The genome appears to be segmented, with regions of dense gene clustering such as the major histocompatibility complex and other regions which are apparently sparse in terms of genes.

A battery of technologies and strategies has now been developed to deal with analysis of the difficult terrain of the human genome. The underlying method used successfully so far in the HGP is to construct a series of maps which serve different functions and act at different levels of resolution all the way down to the DNA sequence. These maps can be cross-referenced because they contain common features or landmarks which are experimentally distinguishable (Fig 1).

Types of map

The genetic map that provides access to the positions of disease genes segregating in families uses the recombination events that occur during meiosis to position markers able to distinguish different copies of the same locus (ie polymorphic), for instance, microsatellites.

A relatively new type of map, known as the 'transcript map', positions a series of markers which tag expressed sequences or genes. This map utilises the technique of radiation hybrid mapping, and can position these expressed sequence tags (ESTs) as well as the genetic microsatellite markers. This, in a sense, gives the positional cloners what they want, which is a map of candidate genes positioned relative to the genetic markers. However (for reasons discussed later), the transcript map made by these approaches can never be complete, and access must be gained to cloned DNA itself in the regions between the genetic markers. This is achieved by making maps of overlapping clones, physical maps or contig maps.

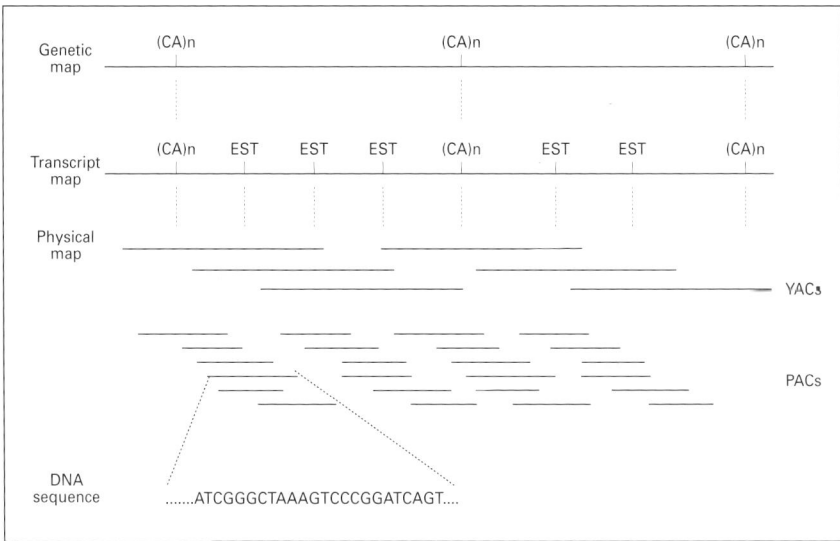

Fig 1. *The hierarchy of genome maps.* Interconnected maps of the human genome using different techniques are connected through common landmarks to form the human genome project product. Horizontal lines represent the continuity of the map for genetic and transcript maps, and the cloned genomic DNA for physical maps, either yeast artificial chromosomes (YACs) or P1-derived artificial chromosomes (PACs), as indicated ((CA)n = polymorphic microsatellite marker; EST = expressed sequence tag).

These physical clone maps can provide the substrate to determine directly the DNA sequence of the human chromosomes. Each map is linked to the others because the markers used are common to each map and their DNA sequence is known.

Human genome project progress

Progress in the HGP may be summarised as follows:

High-resolution genetic map

The high-resolution genetic map of the human genome has been completed.[9] It consists of over 5,000 polymerase chain reaction amplifiable microsatellite markers, positioned at a mean interval of 1.6 cM. This allows a monogenic genetic disease to be mapped to a relatively small physical region of the genome (ca 1–2 Mb). The genetic map can be integrated with the physical and transcript maps, for which it serves as the scaffold.

Expressed sequence tagging

The human genes expressed in a specific tissue can be characterised by short sequences from randomly chosen cDNA clones (the ESTs). The collection of ESTs samples the population of expressed human genes (Fig 2). The sequence reads can come from both the head and tail of the clones because of the nature of cDNA clones. The majority of the reads, however, come from so-called 3' primed cDNA libraries which give a set of sequences from different clones at the 3' end which are overlapping, and a set of sequences from the 5' end which may or may not be overlapping. Large-scale sequencing of these ESTs has placed more than 500,000 ESTs into the public domain. Computer analysis to identify ESTs that overlap each other, and therefore tag the same gene (clustering), suggests that this represents about 42,000 genes.[10] However, transcripts which occur at very low levels, at specific times in development or in specific tissues may not be in these EST collections. It is also clear that a single gene may be represented by more than one cluster and, conversely, multigene families may not be split into different clusters. Thus, a complete resolution of the set of human genes will require the genome sequence.

The transcript map

Substantial parts of the EST-based human gene sets have been placed on a map of the human chromosomes by radiation hybrid mapping to form the so-called transcript map.[10] This map allows

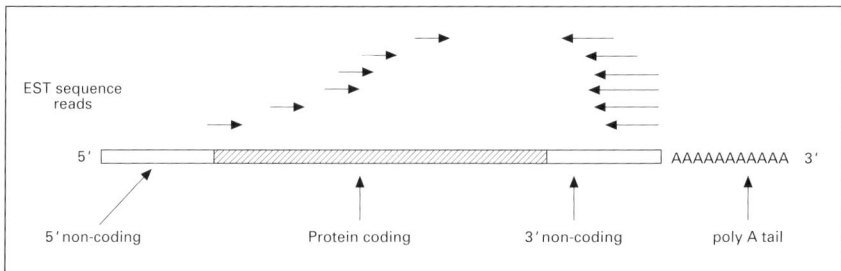

Fig 2. *The structure of a eukaryote mRNA and expressed sequence tags (ESTs).* The open box represents an mRNA transcript, the hashed region corresponding to the open reading frame that is translated. The arrows indicate the positions of a series of single-pass sequence reads derived from arbitrarily picked cDNA clones which each contain a DNA copy (cDNA) of the mRNA transcript, the ESTs.

the geneticist to go from a mapped disease locus to a series of candidate genes in that region (the positional candidate gene approach). At the most recent count, approximately 30,000 gene sequences from a non-redundant EST collection have been positioned relative to each other and the markers of the genetic map (P Deloukas; personal communication).

Yeast artificial chromosome maps

To gain access to all the genomic DNA, including all genes and their control elements, and to elucidate the gene structures, the DNA must be cloned in suitable vectors to produce a physical clone map. All but 10% of the genome has been cloned and ordered in yeast artificial chromosome (YAC) vectors. High-resolution YAC maps are available for chromosomes 3, 4, 7, 12, 16, 19, 21, 22, X and Y (eg see Ref 11). However, because of problems with the fidelity of individual YAC clones and of obtaining large amounts of the cloned DNA free of host yeast cell chromosomes, YACs are not the ideal system for genome sequencing and some other experiments. Hence, 'sequence-ready' maps in cosmids, bacterial artificial chromosomes and P1-derived artificial chromosomes are now being constructed. Substantial coverage is available for some chromosomes (eg 1, 6, 7, 11, 16, 19, 22, X), and this is being extended to all chromosomes to supply the human genome sequencing effort.[12]

Why sequence genomes?

Encoded in the DNA sequence is the complete picture of the genetic complement of an organism, including the genes, their regulatory signals and their relationship to each other on the chromosomes and to the signals used by the transcription and replication apparatuses. Possession of the complete DNA sequence places all the information on a single metric. Moreover, it is only with the complete sequence of a genome that it will be known that nothing has been missed, since other methods to obtain genes in the genome can only sample and are subject to bias.

The experience from sequencing the *S. cerevisiae* genome is informative in this respect. *S. cerevisiae* is an experimental organism about which a great deal was learnt from experimentation over many years, but when the complete sequence was published it became clear that more than half the genes were unknown previously.[13] Sequencing thus provided a whole new way of looking at this organism, and led to new approaches to studying it, such as systematic knock-out of genes predicted from the sequence.

With advances in technology, sequencing – rather than piece-meal approaches – may become the most efficient method of find-ing all the genes in a genome. This is certainly already true for microbes and microbial pathogens whose genomes are well within the scope of current technology and for which the complete sequence can be obtained relatively quickly and easily. The com-plete sequence of a microbial genome gives the full set of genes that define its life cycle and pathogenesis, and instantly produces a whole host of potential drug targets. At least 47 microbial genomes and 17 eukaryote genomes are being, or have already been, sequenced (Table 1 lists genomes that have been completely sequenced).

Human genome sequencing

There are significant differences between genomic sequencing for small genomes and large genomes such as the human genome. The 200-fold difference in the size of the human genome and that of the yeast *S. cerevisiae* makes determining the human genomic sequence a much greater technical and logistical problem. In addi-tion, the genes of bacteria and lower eukaryotes such as *S. cerevisiae* are small, relatively easy to find and have little splicing. From the *S. cerevisiae* sequence it was possible to identify 6,000 open reading frames of 100 codons or larger encoding about 5,800 proteins.[13] Human genes, however, are highly segmented, being spliced together from many small exons, and can often span large genomic regions, even up to 2 Mb, which makes them much

Table 1. Genomes already fully sequenced (adapted from Ref 14).

Genome	Size (kb)
Mycoplasma genitalium	580
Mycoplasma pneumoniae	816
Methanococcus jannaschii	1,665
Helicobacter pylori	1,668
Haemophilus influenzae	1,830
Synechocystis sp.	3,570
Escherichia coli	4,640
Saccharomyces cerevisiae	12,068

harder to identify from the DNA sequence alone without other supporting evidence. Taken together, the difficulty of finding human genes and the size of the genome make determining and interpreting the human genome sequence much harder than for the small genomes.

Human genome sequencing is under way. There are currently 150 Mb of human genomic sequence in the international databases, or 5% of the genome.[15] This is a somewhat inflated percentage, both because of redundancy and because more than one-third of this sequence is precompletion. A true estimate of the genome sequenced would be 2–3%. The progress varies dramatically by chromosome: for chromosomes 7, 22 and X more than 8 Mb of each is already completed and in the databases, while chromosome 18 has less than 100 kb. This reflects the fact that the major sequencing centres have active genomic sequencing efforts organised by chromosome; as these chromosomes get nearer completion, attention will turn to the other chromosomes. Overall, taking into account an extrapolated acceleration in sequencing rate, the current progress is consistent with an expected finishing date of 2006.[15]

The human genome project and human genetic disease

With the improvements in technology and the increased rate of systematic human genome sequencing, it is interesting to ask whether any effect has yet been felt in the area of human genetic disease. Two recent examples which have demonstrated that genomic sequencing can play a major role point to an increased role in the future:

- In a common disease, *hereditary haemochromatosis*, genomic sequencing of the 250 kb region identical by descent in 85% of patient chromosomes, identified a gene with an inactivating missense mutation homozygous in 83% of patients.[16]
- In a much rarer disorder, *Werner's syndrome*, a putative helicase was identified in the candidate region on 8p12 by genomic sequencing with a homozygous frameshift mutation in 60% of Japanese patients.[17]

Interestingly, both these projects involved a major participation from the private sector in the form of small biotech companies, who were able to marshal the resources for a significant genomic sequencing effort, but at the same time be very directed in their targets. Systematic human genome sequencing cannot necessarily be so directed and still be efficient, but these examples perhaps give a glimpse of how genomic sequencing is becoming a tool for positional cloning.

Conclusion

The complete sequence of the human genome will be a permanent resource for biology and medicine. Current trends in the HGP suggest that the sequence will be completed within the next 10 years. So far, the impact of human genome sequencing has been relatively confined but, as the pace quickens, the use of sequence information in human genetics will surely become all pervading. Are we ready?

Acknowledgements

Thanks are expressed to all members of the staff of the Sanger Centre for their help and support; in particular, to Stephan Beck for the preprint of Ref 15, and John Collins, Andy Mungall, Charlotte Cole, David Bentley and Luc Smink for helpful comments on the manuscript. The author is supported by the Wellcome Trust

References

1 Bishop JE, Waldholz M. *Genome: the story of the most astonishing scientific adventure of our time – the attempt to map all the genes in the human body.* New York: Simon and Schuster, 1990.

2 White CS. An interview with Dr Francis Collins. *Carolina Tips* 1995; **58**: 2. (Also available from *Carolina Tips* on-line at http://www.carosci.com/tips/mar95/genome.html)

3 Kitcher P. *The lives to come. The genetic revolution and human possibilities.* New York: Simon and Schuster, 1996.

4 Marshall E. A strategy for sequencing the genome 5 years early. *Science* 1995; **267**: 783–4.

5 US Department of Health and Human Service, US Department of Energy. *Understanding our genetic inheritance. The US human genome project: the first five years.* Bethesda, MD: National Institutes of Health Publication, 1990, No. 90–1590.

6 McKusick VA. The human genome organisation; history, purposes and membership. *Genomics* 1995; **5**: 385–7. http://www.gdb.org/hugo

7 *Summary of the report of the second international strategy meeting on human genome sequencing.* http://www.gdb.org/hugo/bermuda2.htm

8 Fields C, Adams MD, White O, Venter JC. How many genes in the human genome? *Nature Genetics* 1994; **7**: 345–6.

9 Dib C, Faure S, Fizames C, Samson D, *et al.* A comprehensive genetic map of the human genome based on 5,264 microsatellites. *Nature* 1996; **380**: 152–4.

10 Schuler GD, Boguski MS, Stewart EA, Stein LD, *et al.* A gene map of the human genome. *Science* 1996; **274**: 540–6.

11 The genome directory. *Nature* 1995; **377** (Suppl): 1–379.

12 *The Sanger Centre Home Page.* http://www.sanger.ac.uk/. for chromosome 1, 6, 20, 22 and X.

13 The yeast genome directory. *Nature* 1997; **387** (Suppl): 1–105.

14 Doolittle RF. A bug with excess gastric avidity. *Nature* 1997; **388**: 515–6.

15 Beck S, Sterk P. Genome-scale DNA sequencing: where are we? *Current Opinion in Biotechnology* 1998; **9**: 116–20.

16 Feder JN, Gnirke A, Thomas W, Tsuchihashi Z, *et al.* A novel MHC class I-like gene is mutated in patients with hereditary haemochromatosis. *Nature Genetics* 1996; **13**: 399–408.

17 Yu CE, Oshima J, Fu YH, Wijsman EM, *et al.* Positional cloning of the Werner's syndrome gene. *Science* 1996; **272**: 258–62.

Part 2

A spectrum of single gene disorders – an update

4 | Cystic fibrosis

Eric Alton
Imperial College School of Medicine,
National Heart and Lung Institute, London

Pathophysiology

Cystic fibrosis (CF), an autosomal recessively inherited disease affecting approximately one in 2,000 of the Caucasian population, is the commonest lethal inherited disease in the western world. It is characterised by the presence of viscous secretions in a number of organs, particularly the lung. A cycle of respiratory inflammation and infection is responsible for most of the morbidity and mortality seen in this disease. The basic abnormality centres around the CF gene on chromosome 7 producing the CF transmembrane conductance regulator (CFTR) protein.[1] CFTR functions as a chloride channel in the apical membrane of a number of hollow epithelial-lined organs such as the intestinal and respiratory tract.[2] Its physiological role is unknown, but may relate to water movement. In CF subjects, the absence of chloride secretion from the cell on to the mucosal surface of the airways may lead to a concomitant reduction in water flux, and thus to a relative dehydration of the airway surface fluid. This impairs mucociliary clearance, the principal defence mechanism in the lung, leading to retention of bacteria and inhaled particles, and then respiratory infection and respiratory failure.

Some other hypotheses as to how mutant CFTR may cause lung disease have recently been suggested. Several groups have identified that *Pseudomonas aeruginosa*, the commonest pathogen in CF, binds specifically to the surface of respiratory epithelial cells through the asialo GM-1 receptor. It is clear that there is an increased number of these receptors in respiratory epithelial cells in CF, and *CFTR* gene transfer into these cells corrects this abnormality towards normal levels.[3] A further interesting hypothesis relates to the production by the respiratory epithelium of antibiotic-like molecules (defensins, lactoferrin, lysozyme) which turn out to be salt-sensitive with respect to their function. Several studies have suggested that CF airway fluid may contain altered concentrations of salt, related in turn to the ion transport abnormalities, so this may provide a further link between the chloride defect and the pathogenesis of lung disease.

Gene therapy

Preclinical studies

One obvious solution to the condition is to replace the mutant CFTR with a normal copy of the *CFTR* gene. This was first demonstrated to be successful *in vitro*,[4,5] and the advent of CF animal models[6] provided the opportunity to test this *in vivo*. Two groups simultaneously reported that cationic liposome-mediated human *CFTR* gene delivery to the lungs of CF mice was able, at least in part, to correct the basic abnormality in chloride transport.[7,8] Our study demonstrated the feasibility of this using a conventional jet nebuliser, but it is important to note the marked variability in the degree of correction. Some animals showed complete correction whilst others showed no change. Importantly, no safety problems were encountered in either study. These and other studies of liposome-mediated transfer of reporter genes to non-human primates paved the way for human studies.

Clinical studies of liposome-mediated gene transfer

On the basis of this animal work, a study of cationic liposome-mediated gene transfer to the nasal epithelium of CF subjects was undertaken using the liposome DC-CHOL:DOPE.[9] Nasal application was chosen because the nose also demonstrates the basic underlying ion transport defect and provides easier access both for administration and for measurements. Also, it is clearly preferable to assess safety issues in the nose rather than in the lungs. Application was via a commercially available pump spray producing an aerosol of mass median diameter approximately 60 µm. Gene transfer was studied in 15 CF subjects with the commonest mutation ΔF508. Because of the theoretical risk of gene transfer to the gonads, male patients were studied – male CF patients are infertile, so this would circumvent the problem.

Subjects were divided into five groups each of three. Patients in three of the groups were given one of the following doses:

- low dose DNA (10 µg per nostril),
- medium dose (100 µg per nostril), or
- high dose (300 µg per nostril).

The two liposome control groups received liposome equivalent to the 100 µg or 300 µg doses. The study protocol was double-blind and placebo-controlled.

The major goals of the study were to assess safety and whether gene transfer could be achieved. For safety, routine clinical parameters were studied including radiographic changes, blood tests and lung function. A nasal biopsy was taken on day 4, the time at which maximal gene transfer was expected. Biopsy samples were studied in a blinded fashion by an experienced histopathologist. To assess efficiency of gene transfer, vector-specific reverse transcriptase polymerase chain reaction (RT-PCR) from the nasal biopsy was studied (to assess whether the exogenous applied DNA had been transcribed to mRNA). Nasal potential difference measurements (electrophysiological abnormalities) were taken on each of the days on which the patients were assessed.

Results. There were no abnormal clinical events, no abnormalities on the chest X-ray or blood tests, and no differences in the biopsy results between the placebo and *CFTR* gene-treated patients. With regard to the efficacy of gene transfer, vector specific RT-PCR showed the presence of both DNA and mRNA in five of eight available biopsies in treated patients. In terms of the key parameter of functional correction, overall there was an increase of approximately 20% in the chloride response on day 3 following gene transfer ($p < 0.05$) compared to baseline, but this response had completely disappeared by day 7. Some subjects showed virtually complete correction of the chloride response whilst others showed none, in keeping with the variability noted in the animal studies.

Later clinical studies. Subsequent to this study, a number of other liposome-mediated trials have been undertaken both in the UK and the US, and also some studies using adenoviral-mediated gene transfer. The impression is emerging that functional correction of the basic ion transport defect with cationic liposome-mediated gene transfer is as efficient as with adenoviral-mediated gene transfer,[10-12] at least to the nasal epithelium. Neither gene transfer system has apparently produced a major safety issue with respect to the nasal epithelium.

Lung studies

Clearly, the aim of these studies is to demonstrate proof of principle within the lungs rather than in the nasal epithelium of CF subjects. One adenoviral-mediated transfer study[11] has shown the presence of CFTR protein in cells from one of four patients following aerosolisation. A second study from Transgene[13] (France) detected *CFTR* mRNA in one of six patients and CFTR protein in two of six patients, again following aerosolisation.

To date, no study has addressed the issue of liposome-mediated gene transfer to the lungs of CF patients. We have therefore undertaken a programme of work to establish such a trial, first undertaking some preclinical studies to optimise expression. The feasibility of administering the DNA liposome complexes by nebulisation was demonstrated using a clinically relevant nebuliser. No assays of CFTR function that could be used in the lungs have yet been reported. We have now developed a technique for measuring lower airway potential difference via a fibreoptic bronchoscope, and also an *ex vivo* assay using a fluorescent marker of chloride transport in cells obtained by brushing at bronchoscopy. A laboratory-based assay has also been developed for measuring the enhanced binding of *P. aeruginosa* to CF cells, again obtained at brushing.

No study had previously demonstrated the safety of cationic liposomes nebulised into the lungs, so we have recently completed a study assessing the safety of the lipid to be used in the CF study in 15 normal volunteers in a dose escalation manner. No toxicological problems were encountered.

On the basis of these studies, we have recently completed a double-blind, placebo-controlled study in 16 CF subjects, nebulising the *CFTR* DNA complexed to the cationic liposome lipid #67 (Genzyme Corporation, US). The results of this study will be discussed in Chapter 18.

Conclusions

It is clear that proof of principle of gene transfer either through cationic liposomes or adenoviruses both to the upper and lower respiratory tract has now been achieved. However, a number of key questions remain, including:

1   Has gene transfer been achieved in the appropriate cell population within the airways?
2   Has a sufficient level of gene transfer, and hence correction of the basic defect, been achieved?

3 Does this level relate to the number of cells transfected or to the level of correction within certain cells where gene transfer has been achieved or, more likely, to a combination of both?

Most research groups would suggest that gene transfer efficiency will need further augmentation before Phase III clinical studies should be undertaken. This may necessitate further modification of vector systems, but it is more probable that efforts should now be placed on the cellular barriers to efficient gene transfer and on attempts to understand how these can be modified. Given the relatively short time-scale for gene therapy studies so far undertaken, progress has been steady and encouraging.

References

1 Riordan JR, Rommens JM, Kerem B, Alon N, *et al.* Identification of the cystic fibrosis gene: cloning and characterization of complementary DNA. *Science* 1989; **245**: 1066–73.

2 Welsh MJ. Abnormal regulation of ion channels in cystic fibrosis epithelia. *FASEB Journal* 1990; **4**: 2718–25.

3 Davies JC, Stern M, Dewar A, Caplen NJ, *et al.* CFTR gene therapy reduces the binding of *Pseudomonas aeruginosa* to cystic fibrosis respiratory epithelium. *American Journal of Cellular and Molecular Biology* 1997; **16**: 657–63.

4 Drumm ML, Pope HA, Cliff WH, Rommens JM, *et al.* Correction of the cystic fibrosis defect in vitro by retrovirus-mediated gene transfer. *Cell* 1990; **62**: 1227–33.

5 Rich DP, Gregory RJ, Anderson MP, Manavaln P, *et al.* Effect of deleting the R domain on CFTR-generated chloride channels. *Science* 1991; **253**: 205–7.

6 Dorin JR, Alson EW, Porteous DG. Mouse models for cystic fibrosis. In: Dodge JA, Brock DJH, Widdicombe JH (eds). *Cystic fibrosis – current topics*. Chichester: John Wiley & Sons, 1994: 3–31.

7 Hyde SC, Gill DR, Higgins CF, Trezise AE, *et al.* Correction of the ion transport defect in cystic fibrosis transgenic mice by gene therapy. *Nature* 1993; **362**: 250–5.

8 Alton EW, Middleton PG, Caplen NJ, Smith SN, *et al.* Non-invasive liposome-mediated gene delivery can correct the ion transport defect in cystic fibrosis mutant mice. *Nature Genetics* 1993; **5**: 135–42.

9 Caplen NJ, Alton EW, Middleton PG, Dorin JR, *et al.* Liposome-mediated CFTR gene transfer to the nasal epithelium of patients with cystic fibrosis. *Nature Medicine* 1995; **1**: 39–46.

10 Zabner J, Conture LA, Gregory RJ, Graham SM, *et al.* Adenovirus-mediated gene transfer transiently corrects the chloride transport defect in nasal epithelia of patients with cystic fibrosis. *Cell* 1993; **75**: 207–16.

11 Crystal RG, McElvaney NG, Rosenfeld MA, Chu CS, *et al.* Administration of an adenovirus containing the human CFTR cDNA to the respiratory tract of individuals with cystic fibrosis. *Nature Genetics* 1994; **8**: 42–51.

12 Knowles MR, Hohneker KW, Zhou Z, Olsen JC, *et al.* A controlled
    study of adenoviral-vector-mediated gene transfer in the nasal epithe-
    lium of patients with cystic fibrosis. *New England Journal of Medicine*
    1995; **333**: 823–31.
13 Bellon G, Michel-Calemard L, Thouvenot D, Jagneaux V, *et al.*
    Aerosol administration of a recombinant adenovirus expression
    CFTR to cystic fibrosis patients. A Phase I clinical trial. *Human Gene
    Therapy* 1997; **8**: 15–25.

5 | X-linked mental retardation

Sarah Bundey
(Late) Professor of Clinical Genetics, University of Birmingham

Prevalence of mental retardation

Mental retardation (MR) may be divided into severe (IQ <50) or mild (IQ 50–70). The latter group is much larger, comprising 2–3% of all children,[1] and has an appreciable polygenic component with a recurrence risk of 20–25%.[2] X-linked genes make little contribution to mild MR.

Severe MR is less common, accounting for about 0.5% of children,[3,4] is more common in males and has a greater genetic component. The size of the contribution by single genes can be assessed in those patients for whom there is a specific diagnosis, and in undiagnosed cases by the recurrence rate in siblings. About 10–15% of all patients are diagnosed cases of single gene disorder, of whom 7–10% have autosomal conditions[5,6] while 5–10% of males have X-linked MR.[6–8]

Recurrence in sibs of patients with undiagnosed causes for their MR varies with the clinical picture, being lower in children with accompanying features, such as epilepsy and cerebral palsy, and highest in the sibs of those patients who have no distinctive clinical features and whose head circumferences are in the normal range. Children with 'non-specific' MR (NSMR) account for only 14% of all severely retarded children.[9] Their recurrence risks are 9–11% for the brothers of male index patients and 5–6% for their sisters and for the sibs of female index patients.[10,11] These figures suggest that one-quarter of such children have an autosomal recessive disorder with a one in four risk of recurrence for sibs, and that one-tenth of males have an X-linked disorder, with a risk of one in two to one in three for affected brothers.

Combining all these figures, the prevalence of the different single gene disorders which give rise to severe MR can be estimated (Table 1).

Table 1. Approximate prevalence of conditions giving rise to severe mental retardation.

Condition	Girls	Boys	Total
All causes	1/232	1/175	1/200
All autosomal conditions	1/4,000	1/4,000	1/4,000
All X-linked conditions	Very few	1/1,000	1/2,000

Syndromic X-linked mental retardation

The 50–60 examples of syndromic X-linked mental retardation (XLMR) syndromes accompanied by distinguishing features have been summarised by Lubs *et al.*[12]

Xp21 muscular dystrophy

It has been known for many years that Duchenne muscular dystrophy may present with MR,[13] and paediatricians are aware that they must look for large calves and raised creatine kinase (CK) levels in boys with unexplained developmental delay. It has only recently become apparent, however, that milder forms of Xp21 muscular dystrophy (the Becker type) may present with mild MR and emotional and behavioural problems. Four males aged 15, 17, 19 and 42 were described by North *et al.*[14] They presented with mild MR and psychiatric disorder; none had muscle weakness, but all had raised CK levels and evidence of a dystrophinopathy on muscle biopsy.

Mental retardation with haemoglobin-H disease

One of the most interesting XLMR syndromes is that of ATR-X, first recognised in three retarded northern European boys who also had haemoglobin-H disease, a haemoglobinopathy associated with α-thalassaemia in which tetrameres of β-globin accumulate in red cells.[15] Studies of further patients showed that they could be divided into two groups:

• patients with a terminal deletion of 16p (which includes the α-globin genes) associated with a rather variable phenotype; and
• patients with a more consistent phenotype, no deletion of chromosome 16, normal α-globin genes and X-linked inheritance.

The second condition is called ATR-X, and its phenotype includes severe MR, a distinctive facies: telecanthus, epicanthic folds, flat nasal bridge, mid-facial hypoplasia, small nose, anteverted nares, full lips, a protruding tongue, with small, simple and low set ears, and abnormally spaced teeth. The head circumference is less than the 30th centile, and genital abnormalities are common (eg cryptorchidism, small penis and testes, and hypospadias). There may also be a wide range of minor skeletal abnormalities.[16] The diagnosis is made by finding H bodies in circulating red cells. The haematological findings in the ATR-X syndrome are not explained by any abnormality of α-globin genes, but their transcription is reduced. All patients so far have had the XY constitution and many have X-linked pedigrees.

The action of the gene for ATR-X. Gibbons *et al*[17] have demonstrated that the causative gene (*XH2*) belongs to a super family of helicase proteins. Other proteins in this group are involved in recombination, DNA excision repair, transcription and segregation of mitotic chromosomes.[17] This protein for ATR-X has been characterised as having:

• a zinc-finger domain in which two-thirds of the mutations occur;
• a domain that probably interacts with HP1, a chromatin protein;
• a helicase domain; and
• a region in which mutations are associated with sex reversal.[18]

The authors suggest that the ATR-X protein is involved with distant effects on the transcription of genes, such as the α-globin genes, through an effect mediated by binding to chromatin proteins. It occurs if the amount of ATR-X protein is reduced to 30% or less.

It is interesting that another X linked condition, the Juberg-Marsidi syndrome which produces severe MR, growth failure, deafness, hypogenitalism and early death, is also due to mutations in the XH2 gene.[19] This is another example of X-linked conditions due to mutations in the same X-linked gene having different phenotypes (Table 2).

The fragile-X syndrome

The fragile-X syndrome probably accounts for about one-third of all XLMR conditions and for 3–4% of all retarded males, and has a

Table 2. XL genes in which different mutations give rise to different phenotypes, some of which are associated with mental retardation.

Gene	Location	Phenotype	Ref
Dystrophin	Xp21	Duchenne muscular dystrophy	13
		Becker muscular dystrophy	14
NDP	Xp11	Norrie disease	20
		Exudative retinopathy	21
XH2	Xq12	ATR-X	17
		Juberg-Marsidi syndrome	19
MNK	Xq13	Menkes disease	22
		Mild Menkes disease	23
		Occipital horn syndrome	23
PLP	Xq21	Pelizaeus-Merzbacher disease	24
		Complicated spastic paraplegia	25
		Pure spastic paraplegia	26
L1CAM	Xq28	Spastic paraplegia and mental retardation	27
		Hydrocephalus	28

prevalence of $1/4,000–1/5,000$.[29,30] When first described, it was noteworthy for unusual features about its inheritance, which have now become explicable following the cloning of the fragile-X gene (the *FMR1* gene) in May 1991. The mutation that explains nearly all cases of the fragile-X syndrome consists of an increased number of CGG repeats upstream of the *FMR1* gene. An expansion to over 200 repeats results in methylation of the *FMR1* gene, which then fails to be transcribed. The fragile-X phenotype is thus due to total lack of the gene product. The clinical features are non-specific:

- IQ: 35–70;
- head circumference above the 50th centile;
- post-pubertal testicular size over the 50th centile; and
- the skin may be soft and pliant.

One unusual feature is that female carriers of the fragile-X tend to have premature menopause (6–8 years earlier than the general population),[31] and dizygotic twinning is more common than expected among their offspring.

The CGG repeat in the fragile-X syndrome. Normally there are 0–50 CGG repeats on each X chromosome, and these are stable when transmitted. A range of repeats from 50 to 200 indicates a 'premutation', while repeats numbering over 200 have path-ological consequences with methylation and switching off of the *FMR1* gene. All males with more than 200 repeats and half the females with more than 200 repeats are retarded. The number of repeats expands only in female meiosis, and the degree of in-stability (ie change of length) varies with the absolute length of the repeat in the mother. It is interesting that there is a selection against the appearance of more than 200 repeats in the sperm, and males with more than 200 repeats in their blood have less than 200 repeats in their sperm.

The repeats can be measured by polymerase chain reaction (PCR), so DNA tests have superseded chromosome tests. PCR analysis can detect affected patients and carriers of premutations, and can also be used for prenatal diagnosis.

Inheritance patterns. There are several different inheritance patterns according to the sex of the individual and whether there is a mutation or a premutation:

- A male with a full mutation will have sperm containing only premutations; all his daughters will be mentally normal but will be premutation carriers.
- A male with a premutation will pass this on unchanged to his daughters who will be clinically healthy but run the risk of having children with the full mutation.
- A female with a full mutation will have a 50% chance for each son to be retarded, and a 50% chance for each daughter to carry the full mutation but only half will be retarded. Thus, half her sons and three-quarters of her daughters will be mentally normal.
- For a female with a premutation, the situation is more complicated. She may have:
  - retarded sons with a full mutation (due to expansion during meiosis),
  - healthy sons who carry a normal sized repeat,
  - healthy sons who are premutation carriers,
  - daughters with the full mutation (half of whom will be mentally retarded), or
  - healthy daughters who carry a normal sized repeat or are premutation carriers.

The precise risk for these events depends on the size of the mother's premutation. For expansions of 80 repeats or less, the risk of a carrier having a retarded child is low, perhaps of the order of 1%. Expansions of 130 repeats or over confer a risk of 40–50% for a son to be retarded and 20–25% for a daughter to be retarded, with smaller risks for children to be premutation carriers. The genetic risks for carriers with expansions of 80–130 are not known.

When giving genetic counselling, it is important to be honest about the uncertainty as to how likely a premutation is to expand during female meiosis. Prenatal diagnosis is possible, with sizing of the repeats in a fetus, but it is not possible to predict whether or not a female fetus with a full mutation will be mentally retarded.

The action of the FMR1 gene. In the disease state, *FMR1*, the fragile-X gene, produces no protein. In healthy individuals, the protein product (FMRP) is particularly abundant in the neurones of the brain and spermatogonia of the testes, but it also occurs in other tissues.[32] It is associated with ribosomal proteins in the cytoplasm and is thought to impair protein assembly through impaired RNA binding.[33] An autosomal homologue to the *FMR1* gene has been located to chromosome 12q13,[34] and it will be interesting to see whether this is involved in any of the autosomal recessive types of MR.

Other X-linked syndromes

Coffin-Lowry syndrome. A causative gene has been identified in another XLMR syndrome, the Coffin-Lowry syndrome which is quite variable in its manifestations. Essentially, it consists of severe MR with facial dysmorphism, puffy tapering fingers and skeletal deformities.[35] The locus is at Xp22 which led Trivier *et al*[36] to consider the gene for Rsk-2 as a candidate, and indeed they found mutations in some patients. The gene product is a growth factor-regulated protein kinase which is involved in signalling. It acts as a substrate for several transcription factors, and this may be the mechanism whereby it affects development of brain and bone.

Aarskog-Scott syndrome. Another X-linked syndrome in which MR, skeletal abnormality and urogenital abnormalities occur is the Aarskog-Scott syndrome. Its causative gene was cloned by Pasteris *et al* in 1994,[37] and mutations were found in two families. The gene is homologous to several proto-oncogenes involved in the regulation of growth-related signal transduction. It has been proposed that it acts on developing tissue through binding to *RAS* or related proteins, and that its absence significantly affects normal development of brain, bone and the urogenital system.

Genetic counselling with an X-linked pedigree

Genetic counselling is straightforward when there is an X-linked pedigree: the daughters and mothers of affected males will all be carriers, and their sisters will have a one in two chance of being affected. If mutation analysis is not possible, prenatal prediction of an affected male fetus can usually be carried out using linkage.

Genetic counselling without an X-linked pedigree

In a situation where an affected male has a diagnosable condition, but is the only affected case in the family, the decision has to be made about whether or not the mother is a carrier. In some conditions, like the Coffin-Lowry syndrome,[35] there are often only minor features of the carrier state in females but their absence does not rule out carrier status. It is usually considered that one-third of affected boys with an X-linked condition that precludes procreation are affected by new mutations, and that in two-thirds of instances their mothers are carriers – an assumption based on equal mutation rates in oogenesis and spermatogenesis. However, this pattern will not be true for all X-linked conditions (the fragile-X syndrome being one obvious exception) because, as mentioned earlier, all mothers are carriers of either premutations or full mutations.

Non-specific mental retardation

The category of NSMR includes those children who are mentally retarded but lack distinctive symptoms or signs. They lack significant dysmorphic features, their head circumferences are in the normal range, they do not suffer from epilepsy or have abnormal neurological signs. The fragile-X syndrome may be included under this heading because many affected children lack distinctive features,[8] but some authors (eg Lubs *et al*[12]) place it in the syndrome category. In any case, the condition is diagnosable through molecular tests, and indeed blood samples from all children, male or female, who present with NSMR should undergo molecular testing at the DNA laboratory for the fragile-X mutation, and consideration also be given to measuring the levels of CK and looking for H inclusions in red cells.

There are 41 families in the literature with NSMR and no fragile-X mutation, and with sufficient affected family members to give useful results on linkage analysis.[12] Some of these families may be affected by different mutations in the same gene. There are likely to be at least 10–12 separate loci to account for these families. It will be interesting to discover in due course what the genes are and what they do. In the meantime, linked markers may be used for genetic counselling if there are several affected males; where there are not, empirical recurrence risks must be used.

Genetic counselling with unknown mode of inheritance

One male or two affected brothers with non-specific mental retardation. The most difficult genetic counselling situations are those in which there is one male patient or two affected brothers who have an undiagnosed type of severe NSMR – a small category, but it causes problems. An important question for their sisters is whether the males have an X-linked condition; if this is the case, the former may be at risk of having similarly affected sons.

One set of data for assessing the risk of one or two males having an X-linked condition comes from the study of Herbst and Miller[7] who analysed the British Columbia Health Surveillance Registry (BCHSR) for children with NSMR of all severities born between 1950 and 1969. There were 35 sibships with two or more affected sisters and 107 sibships with two or more affected brothers, implying that the excess of 72 sibships had X-linked MR. Estimates were then made about the number of carrier mothers likely to be in the population, and it was finally estimated that 27% of males with NSMR of all degrees had an X-linked disorder. About 2–3% would have been mildly retarded[30] and, with improvement in diagnoses, some of these boys would now have a specific label, particularly that of fragile-X syndrome. This means that the percentage of males with X-linked causes for their severe NSMR has to be adjusted downwards. The most helpful way to do this is to use the empirical recurrence risks within families listed at the beginning of this chapter (summarised in Table 3). Probably about 10% of males with NSMR and no affected relatives have an undiagnosed X-linked disorder, giving a 2–5% risk for their sisters being a carrier.

Two or more affected males with non-specific mental retardation. In the case of sibships with two or more affected males with NSMR, it is assumed that such pairs of similarly affected sibs will have a genetic disorder. The data from sib-pairs known to the BCHSR[7] suggest that about one-third will have autosomal recessive disease, and the others one of the forms of X-linked mental retardation, with affected male relatives in the maternal lineage in about half the cases. Therefore,

Table 3. Recurrence risks for families with one or more males affected by non-specific, undiagnosed severe mental retardation.[7,10,11]

	Recurrence in:			
	Brothers (%)	Sisters (%)	Sisters' sons (%)	Ratio AR:XL disease
1 male index patient; no affected relative	9–11*	5–6	2–5	2.5:1
≥2 brothers affected; no other affected relative	34**	17	17	2:1
XL pedigree	50	Low	25	0:1

*made up of risks of 5–6% and 4–5% for autosomal recessive (AR) and X-linked (XL) disease, respectively.
**made up of risks of 17% for both AR ($\frac{2}{3} \times \frac{1}{4}$) and XL disease ($\frac{1}{3} \times \frac{1}{2}$).

if there are two brothers with a similar type of NSMR, without affected uncles or cousins and who test negative with the fragile-X syndrome, their overall chance of having an X-linked form of mental retardation is one in three, and the risk for a sister being a carrier is one in six. These risks are set out in Table 3.

References

1   Birch HG, Richardson SA, Baird D, Horobin G, Illsley R. *Mental subnormality in the community: a clinical and epidemiological study.* Baltimore: Williams & Wilkins, 1970.

2   Bundey S, Thake A, Todd J. The recurrence risks for mild idiopathic mental retardation. *Journal of Medical Genetics* 1989; **26**: 260–6.

3   Penrose LS. A clinical and genetic study of 1,280 cases of mental defect. *Medical Research Council Special Report* No. 229, 1938. (Reprinted by the Institute for Research into Mental and Multiple Handicap, 1975.)

4   Kushlick A, Cox GR. The epidemiology of mental handicap. *Developmental Medicine and Child Neurology* 1973; **15**: 748–59.

5   Gustavson K-H, Hagberg B, Hagberg G, Sars K. Severe mental retardation in a Swedish county. *Neuropadiatrie* 1977; **8**: 293–304.

6   Laxova R, Ridler MAC, Bowes-Bravery M. An etiological survey of the severely retarded Hertfordshire children who were born between January 1, 1965 and December 31, 1967. *American Journal of Medical Genetics* 1967; **1**: 75–86.

7   Herbst DS, Miller JR. Non-specific X-linked mental retardation II: the frequency in British Columbia. *American Journal of Medical Genetics* 1980; **7**: 461–9.

8   Turner G, Robinson H, Laing S, Purvis-Smith S. Preventive screening

for the fragile X syndrome. *New England Journal of Medicine* 1986; **315**: 607–9.

9 Bundey S, Carter CO. Recurrence risks in severe undiagnosed mental deficiency. *Journal of Mental Deficiency Research* 1974; **18**: 115–34.

10 Herbst DS, Baird PA. Sib risks for non-specific mental retardation in British Columbia. *American Journal of Medical Genetics* 1982; **13**: 197–208.

11 Bundey S, Webb TP, Thake A, Todd J. A community study of severe mental retardation in the West Midlands and the importance of the fragile X chromosome in its aetiology. *Journal of Medical Genetics* 1985; **22**: 258–66.

12 Lubs HA, Chiurazzi P, Arena JF, Schwartz C, *et al.* XLMR genes: update 1996. *American Journal of Medical Genetics* 1996; **64**: 147–57.

13 Prosser EJ, Murphy EG, Thompson MW. Intelligence and the gene for Duchenne muscular dystrophy. *Archives of Disease in Childhood* 1969; **44**: 221–30.

14 North KN, Miller G, Iannaccone ST, Clemens PR, *et al.* Cognitive dysfunction as the major presenting feature of Becker's muscular dystrophy. *Neurology* 1996; **46**: 461–5.

15 Weatherall DJ, Higgs DR, Bunch C, Old JM, *et al.* Hemoglobin H disease and mental retardation: a new syndrome or a remarkable coincidence? *New England Journal of Medicine* 1981; **305**: 607–12.

16 Gibbons RJ, Wilkie AOM, Weatherall DJ, Higgs DR. A newly defined X-linked mental retardation syndrome associated with α-thalassaemia. *Journal of Medical Genetics* 1991; **28**: 729–33.

17 Gibbons RJ, Picketts DJ, Villard L, Higgs DR. Mutations in a putative global transcriptional regulator cause X-linked mental retardation with α-thalassaemia (ATR-X) syndrome. *Cell* 1995; **80**: 837–45.

18 Gibbons RJ, Bachoo S, Picketts DJ, Aftimos S, *et al.* Mutations in transcriptional regulator ATRX establish the functional significance of a PHD-like domain. *Nature Genetics* 1997; **17**: 146–8.

19 Villard L, Gecz J, Mattéi JF, Fontes M, *et al.* XNP mutation in a large family with Juberg-Marsidi syndrome. *Nature Genetics* 1996; **12**: 359–60.

20 Chen Z-Y, Battinelli EM, Hendricks RW, Powell JF, *et al.* Norrie disease gene: characterization of deletions and possible function. *Genomics* 1993; **16**: 533–5.

21 Chen Z-Y, Battinelli EM, Fielder A, Bundey S, *et al.* A mutation in the Norrie disease gene (NDP) associated with X-linked familial exudative vitreoretinopathy. *Nature Genetics* 1993; **5**: 180–3.

22 Vulpe C, Levinson B, Whitney S, Packman S, Gitschier J. Isolation of a candidate gene for Menkes disease and evidence that it encodes a copper-transporting ATPase. *Nature Genetics* 1993; **3**: 7–13.

23 Kaler SG, Gallo LK, Proud VK, Percy AK, *et al.* Occipital horn syndrome and a mild Menkes phenotype associated with splice site mutations at the MNK locus. *Nature Genetics* 1994; **8**: 195–202.

24 Geneic S, Abuelo D, Ambler M, Hudson LD. Pelizaeus-Merzbacher disease: an X-linked neurologic disorder of myelin metabolism with a novel mutation in the gene encoding proteolipid protein. *American Journal of Human Genetics* 1989; **45**: 435–42.

25 Kobayashi H, Hoffman EP, Marks HG. The rumpshaker mutation in spastic paraplegia. *Nature Genetics* 1994; **7**: 351–2.

26 Cambi F, Tang X-M, Cordray P, Fain PR, *et al.* Refined genetic mapping and proteolipid protein mutation analysis in X-linked pure hereditary spastic paraplegia. *Neurology* 1996; **46**: 1112–7.

27 Jouet M, Rosenthal A, Armstrong G, MacFarlane J, *et al.* X-linked spastic paraplegia (SPG1), MASA syndrome and X-linked hydrocephalus result from mutations in the L1 gene. *Nature Genetics* 1994; **7**: 402–7.

28 Rosenthal A, Jouet M, Kenwrick S. Aberrant splicing of L1CAM mRNA associated with X-hydrocephalus. *Nature Genetics* 1992; **2**: 107–12.

29 Murray A, Youings S, Dennis N, Latsky L, *et al.* Population screening at the FRAXA and FRAXE loci: molecular analyses of boys with learning difficulties and their mothers. *Human Molecular Genetics* 1996; **5**: 727–35.

30 Morton JE, Bundey S, Webb TP, MacDonald F, *et al.* Fragile X syndrome is less common than previously estimated. *Journal of Medical Genetics* 1997; **34**: 1–5.

31 Partington MW, York-Moore D, Turner GM. Confirmation of early menopause in fragile X carriers. *American Journal of Medical Genetics* 1996; **34**: 370–2.

32 Devys D, Lutz Y, Rouyer N, Bellocq J-P, Mandel J-L. The FMR-1 protein is cytoplasmic, most abundant in neurons and appears normal in carriers of a fragile-X premutation. *Nature Genetics* 1993; **4**: 335–40.

33 Khandjian EW, Corbin F, Woerly S, Rousseau F. The fragile X mental retardation protein is associated with ribosomes. *Nature Genetics* 1996; **12**: 91–3.

34 Siomi MC, Siomi H, Sauer W, Srinivasan S, *et al.* FXR1, an autosomal homolog of the fragile X mental retardation gene. *EMBO Journal* 1995; **14**: 2401–8.

35 Young ID. The Coffin-Lowry syndrome. *Journal of Medical Genetics* 1988; **25**: 344–8.

36 Trivier E, De Cesare D, Jacquot S, Pannetier S, *et al.* Mutations in the kinase Rsk-2 associated with Coffin-Lowry syndrome. *Nature* 1996; **384**: 567–70.

37 Pasteris NG, Cadle A, Logie LJ, Porteous ME, *et al.* Isolation and characterisation of the faciogenital dysplasia (Aarskog-Scott syndrome) gene: a putative Rho/Rac guanine nucleotide exchange factor. *Cell* 1994; **79**: 669–78.

6 | Muscular dystrophies

Peter Lunt
Institute of Child Health,
Bristol Royal Hospital for Sick Children

Molecular research in muscular dystrophies, particularly Duchenne, Becker and myotonic dystrophies, has been at the forefront of genetic research for the past 15 years, often providing the lead for molecular findings in other conditions.[1] Much of this research has been made possible through charity funding from the muscular dystrophy associations, including the Muscular Dystrophy Group of Great Britain.[2]

Knowledge of the human genome enables molecular genetics to assist currently or potentially in the care of muscular dystrophy patients and families through:

- diagnosis,
- prognosis,
- genetic management of families, and
- treatment.

Diagnosis

Diagnosis in muscular dystrophy is made from a combination of:

- clinical history and examination,
- serum chemistry (creatine kinase (CK), lactate),
- electrophysiology (electromyography (EMG), ± nerve conduction study),
- inheritance pattern,
- muscle biopsy (routine and specific immunohistochemical staining), and
- specific mutation detection on DNA.

Clinical presentation

The diagnosis in a four year old boy with pelvic weakness and

Gowers sign, calf hypertrophy, lumbar lordosis, a serum CK above 10,000 iu/l, and an X-linked recessive family history of similar boys requiring a wheelchair by the age of 12 years will undoubtedly be Duchenne muscular dystrophy (DMD), but this is not always the case when such a child presents for the first time in a family. Some forms of autosomal recessive limb-girdle muscular dystrophy (LGMD) (those previously termed severe childhood autosomal recessive muscular dystrophy (SCARMD)) can present with an almost identical clinical picture,[1,3–5] while some of the most severe cases of facioscapulohumeral muscular dystrophy (FSHD) may also have been misdiagnosed initially as the Duchenne type.[6]

Inheritance pattern

The inheritance pattern shown by a particular gene defect depends on whether the gene concerned is on the X chromosome, on one of the 22 autosomes or in mitochondrial DNA, and also on the effect of the particular mutation on the normal action of the encoded protein product. In familial cases, recognition of the inheritance pattern can help establish the diagnosis (summarised for the more common muscular dystrophies in Table 1).

Table 1. Inheritance patterns in the more common muscular dystrophies.

	Dominant	Recessive	X-linked	Maternal
Muscular dystrophy	FSHD Myotonic	LGMD SCARMD Congenital	Duchenne Becker Emery-Dreifuss	
Other neuromuscular disorders				
Congenital myopathy	+	+	+	
SMA	+	++	+/−	
HMSN	++	+	+	
Mitochondrial myopathy+	+	+	+	++

FSHD	= facioscapulohumeral muscular dystrophy
HMSN	= hereditary motor and sensory neuropathy
LGMD	= limb-girdle muscular dystrophy
SCARMD	= severe childhood autosomal recessive muscular dystrophy
SMA	= spinal muscular atrophy

Muscle biopsy

The appearances on a routine haematoxylin and eosin stained muscle biopsy of fibre size variation, internal nuclei, hyalinised fibres, fibre splitting and increased perimyseal connective tissue can establish a diagnosis of muscular dystrophy, but much less reliably the particular type. Genome research has led to the mapping of muscular dystrophy gene loci, and hence to the identification of the encoded gene products.[7] Antibodies raised against these form the basis of specific immunohistochemical stains which are now used on biopsies to define the specific type of dystrophy.

Dystrophin

In DMD, the key to isolation of dystrophin as the gene product came from a boy (BB), described by Francke in 1985[8] who, in addition to DMD and mental retardation, had chronic granulomatous disease, McLeod red cell phenotype (absence of Kell blood group antigen) and retinitis pigmentosa. He had a cytogenetically detectable deletion of Xp21 region, resulting in deletion of contiguous genes in this region of the short arm of the X chromosome – hence his presentation with several different X-linked recessive conditions.

The dystrophin gene, cloned through a particular laboratory technique made possible by this boy's deletion, was indeed located in Xp21; it spans 2 Mb of DNA, and has proved to be one of the largest human genes known.[9] The coding sequence is divided between 78 exons, and in muscle fibres produces an RNA transcript 14 kb long. The large size probably accounts for the high mutation rate and relative prevalence of the condition. Expression of the dystrophin gene is not restricted to muscle, but also occurs in heart, brain and liver. There are now known to be alternative ways to splice the transcribed RNA, and different transcription promoters or splice sites may be used in these other tissues to give slightly different products from the dystrophin gene.[10]

Muscle biopsy confirmation of a clinical diagnosis of DMD now relies on immunostaining showing absence of the dystrophin gene product (Fig 1). Similarly, Becker muscular dystrophy (BMD) is diagnosed from a subtotal loss of dystrophin on immunostain (see Fig 4(c)).

Other muscle proteins

Family studies for genetic linkage in other forms of muscular dystrophy, and in certain other hereditary myopathies, have over the

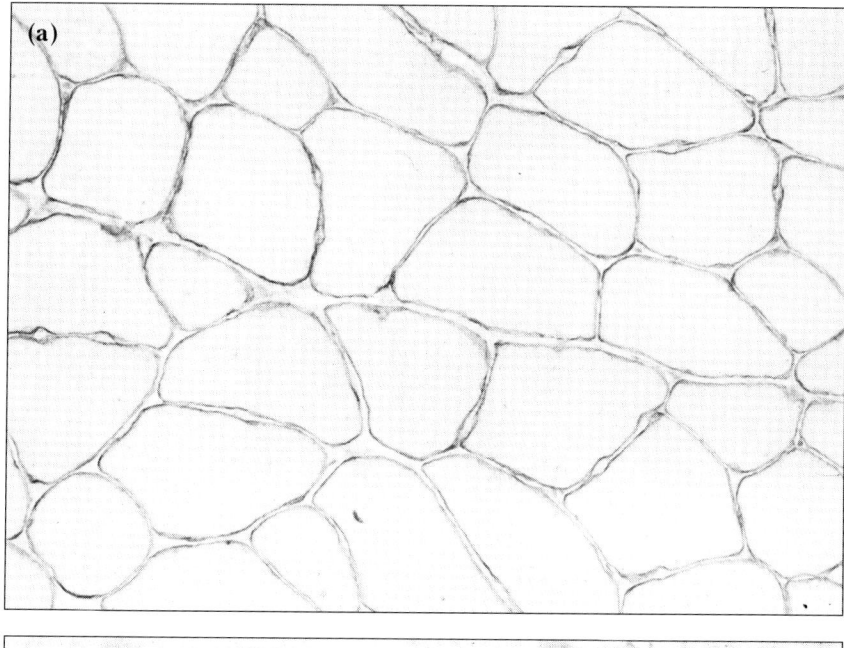

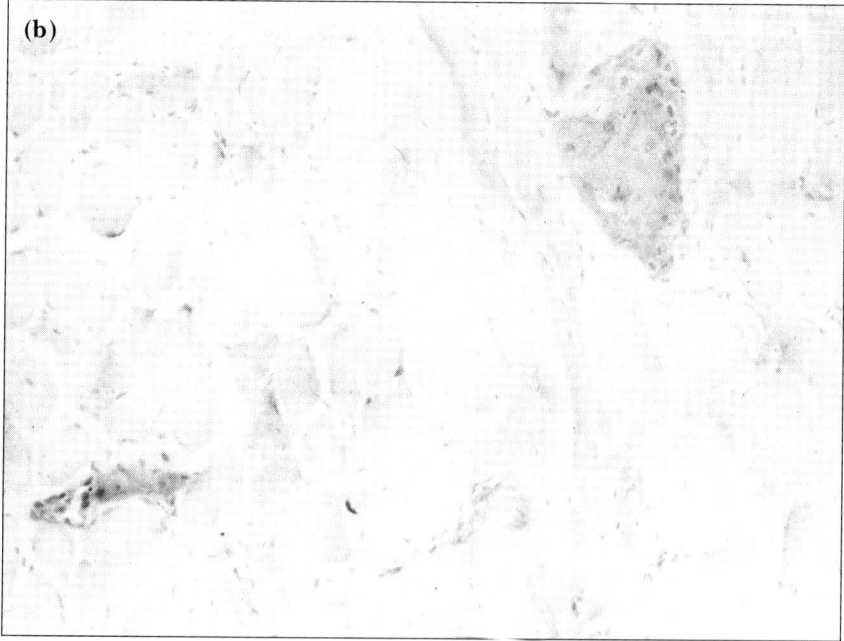

Fig 1. *Muscle biopsies, immunostained with anti-dystrophin Dys-2 antibody:* **(a)** *normal control* – note uniform distribution of dystrophin localised to sub-sarcolemma, with general background features of relatively uniform fibre size and peripherally sited nuclei; **(b)** *4 year old boy with Duchenne muscular dystrophy* – note absence of dystrophin from sarcolemmal region, and general features of increased variation in fibre size and some internal nuclei (reproduced by courtesy of Professor S Love, Bristol).

past few years led to the mapping, cloning and characterisation of the relevant genes.[7] This, paralleled by the direct isolation of muscle structural proteins, has led to the identification of the proteins involved in these disorders and to a model of their anatomical organisation (Fig 2).[11,12] In particular, at least six different genes (and their encoded proteins) can be implicated in families with autosomal recessive forms of LGMD.[3,12] Three (or possibly four) of these code for subunits of the *sarcoglycan complex* which traverses the sarcolemmal membrane. Homozygosity for mutation in the genes encoding the alpha- or gamma-sarcoglycan subunit results in a severe childhood presentation which is clinically indistinguishable from that of DMD, except for the inheritance pattern, and consequent equal sex ratio.[13,14] Although – fortunately for differential diagnosis – such cases are rare in comparison with DMD, they should be particularly suspected in a female index case or where there is parental consanguinity.

Diagnosis of the individual types of LGMD has been made possible through the identification of the proteins involved, and is now achieved primarily from muscle biopsy through immunostaining for these specific proteins. Figure 3 shows a biopsy from a child presenting with a Duchenne-like clinical picture, but diagnosed from the immunostaining pattern as a gamma-sarcoglycanopathy (LGMD2C) with an autosomal recessive inheritance pattern. This was confirmed by subsequent identification in the child's DNA of two mutations in the gamma-sarcoglycan gene.

Immunostaining for *emerin*, which locates to the nuclear membrane (Fig 2), can now provide a confirmatory diagnostic test (possibly from lymphocytes) for X-linked Emery-Dreifuss muscular dystrophy (EDMD),[15,16] characterised clinically by joint contractures, cardiomyopathy, colour blindness and a scapuloperoneal distribution of muscle weakness. Similarly, *merosin* deficiency accounts for 50% of congenital muscular dystrophy, and is diagnosed from immunostaining.[17] LGMD2A, which is prevalent in the Amish, the Basque population and on the Island of Reunion, is of particular interest in being due to an enzyme deficiency (calpain 3) rather than a structural muscle protein.[18]

DNA as a diagnostic test through mutation detection

The detection of mutation in a particular gene in a DNA sample extracted from peripheral blood can be used as a fully specific diagnostic test for the relevant genetic condition. However, the

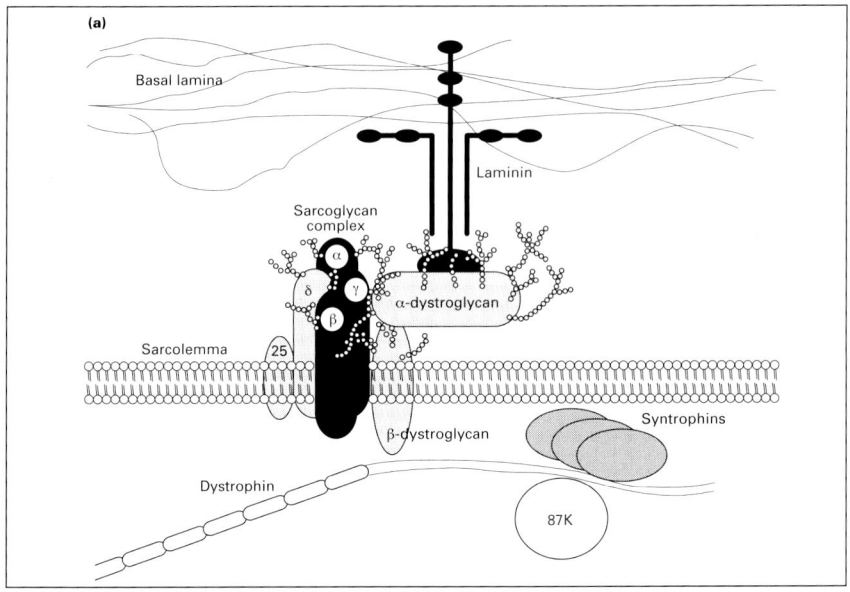

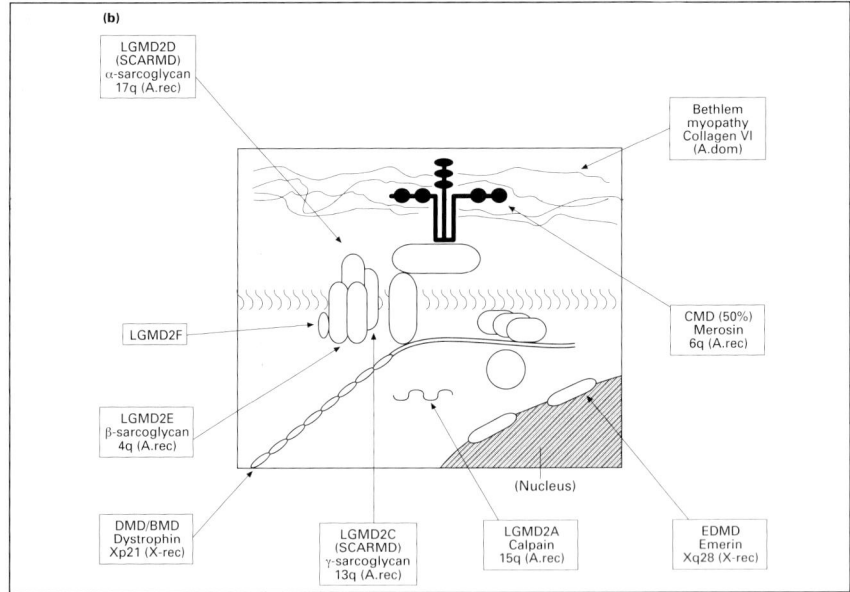

Fig 2. *Muscle proteins involved in muscular dystrophies*: **(a)** *a proposed model of membrane organisation of the dystrophin-glycoprotein complex;*[11] **(b)** *assignment, following gene mapping and cloning, of the protein subunits at fault in individual muscular dystrophies* (A. dom = autosomal dominant; A. rec = autosomal recessive; BMD = Becker muscular dystrophy; CMD = childhood muscular dystrophy; DMD = Duchenne muscular dystrophy; EDMD = Emery-Dreifuss muscular dystrophy; LGMD = limb-girdle muscular dystrophy; SCARMD = severe childhood autosomal recessive muscular dystrophy; X-rec = X (chromosome)-linked recessive).

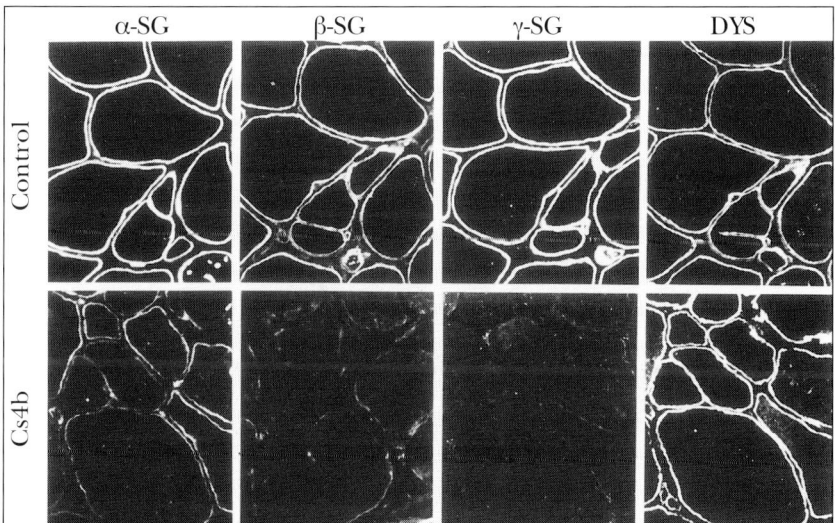

Fig 3. *Limb-girdle muscular dystrophy (LGMD) (severe childhood presentation).*
Muscle biopsy from patient (Cs4b) and control immunostained for alpha-
(α-SG), beta- (β-SG) and gamma-sarcoglycan (γ-SG) and dystrophin
(DYS). Note a moderate reduction from normal of α-SG, a severe reduction of β-SG, and complete absence of γ-SG, while DYS was normal. This
patient had a γ-sarcoglycanopathy (LGMD2C), subsequently confirmed by
finding mutations in the γ-SG gene on chromosome 13q (reproduced by
courtesy of Dr C Sewry, Hammersmith Hospital, London).

search for mutation, if likely to be family-specific or if the gene
under test may not be the appropriate one, is often an involved
labour-intensive process which can be contemplated only as part of
a separately funded research programme. Therefore, currently,
mutation detection can be sufficiently efficient for use in a
diagnostic service setting only if there is a uniform or prevalent
mutation mechanism as the cause of a condition.

Duchenne/Becker muscular dystrophy. In DMD or BMD, 65% of mutations are due to deletion of one or more exons of the dystrophin
gene.[19] Despite its size, the gene can be readily screened to identify
whether any exons are deleted by employing a small number of
multiplex polymerase chain reaction (PCR) analyses which simultaneously amplify several different exons.[20] This has advantages over
muscle biopsy as a confirmatory diagnostic test for Xp21 dystrophy
in those 65% cases both because it requires a much less invasive
procedure (venepuncture) and because of the potential rapidity
with which a result is obtained. Muscle biopsy is nevertheless still

recommended to help differentiate between DMD and BMD, and hence help predict the prognosis.

Facioscapulohumeral muscular dystrophy. Deletion at chromosome region 4q35 in FSHD of an integral number of copies of a tandemly repeated 3.3 kb DNA sequence (which contains a homeodomain) accounts for over 95% of cases.[21,22] Detection of the deletion, and therefore confirmation of diagnosis, is possible in DNA from peripheral blood, but in some cases requires pulse field gel electrophoresis (PFGE) of high molecular weight DNA (and therefore a very fresh blood sample) for distinction from a normal control polymorphism.[22,23]

Myotonic dystrophy. The presence of a significant expansion of a CTG trinucleotide repeat sequence in the myotonic dystrophy (DM) protein kinase gene at 19q13 provides a simple, rapid, highly specific (>99%) and sensitive diagnostic test for the condition. This should now replace all other invasive investigations (including EMG) as the primary and definitive diagnostic test.[24]

Other muscular dystrophies. Mutation detection in other muscular dystrophies, or in the 35% of DMD/BMD without a deletion, requires an individual approach to each family to identify the family-specific mutation. This is beginning to be possible for purposes of genetic counselling once muscle biopsy has shown a patient to have deficiency of a particular muscle protein. However, there must be a greater efficiency or automation of the techniques involved before the search for a family-specific mutation in any one of several possible genes can be contemplated as a primary diagnostic test.

Prognosis

For a given genetic diagnosis, the quantity of gene product detected by specific immunostaining of muscle biopsy or the specific DNA mutation may in some circumstances provide prognostic information. Thus, the distinction of Becker from Duchenne dystrophy is facilitated by finding a reduction in rather than absence of dystrophin immunostain in muscle (Fig 4).[25]

In several muscular dystrophies, correlation can be made at DNA level between genotype and phenotype, allowing some degree of prognostic prediction.

Duchenne/Becker muscular dystrophy. The distinction between deletions

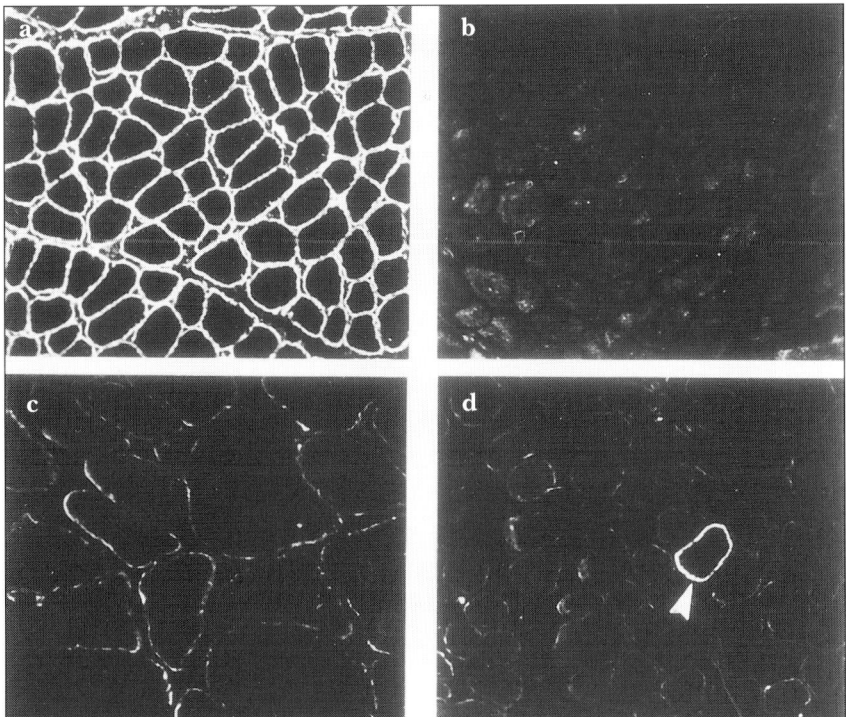

Fig 4. *Dystrophin immunostaining of muscle biopsies from four patients:* (**a**) *normal control;* (**b**) *Duchenne muscular dystrophy (DMD), dystrophin absent;* (**c**) *Becker muscular dystrophy, dystrophin reduced, with uneven patchy staining;* (**d**) *DMD, isolated 'revertant' fibre with immunologically recognisable dystrophin.* (reproduced by courtesy of Dr C Sewry, Hammersmith Hospital, London).

causing DMD or BMD depends not so much on their size, but rather on whether or not they delete a multiple of 3 bp from exon sequences:[26]

- A deletion which shifts the subsequent reading frame (frameshift mutation) will result in the premature encountering of a STOP codon, and therefore in a severe (Duchenne) phenotype.
- A deletion of (3 × n) bp which leaves subsequent codons 'in-frame' will result in a shortened protein product, but one which has both the amino- and carboxy- ends intact, and therefore in a milder (Becker) phenotype (see Fig 5).

Different dystrophin mutations may also have different effects on the alternative transcripts produced in other tissues; for example, it may be that only certain mutations cause associated learning difficulties.[27]

Normal											
	.....	You	Ca**n**	**See**	And	You	Can	Now	Ken	All	......
DMD											
	.....	You	Caa	Ndy	Ouc	Ann	Owk	Ena	Ll..		....
BMD											
	.....	You	Cad	You	Can	Now	Ken	All		....	

Fig 5. *Illustrative effect on the triplet codon reading frame of deletions which do (Becker muscular dystrophy (BMD): 6 base pairs deleted) or do not (Duchenne muscular dystrophy (DMD): 4 base pairs deleted) involve a multiple of three base pairs.*

Myotonic dystrophy. The length of the CTG trinucleotide repeat broadly correlates with clinical severity in DM, the largest expansions being found in patients with congenital onset. The CTG repeat also tends to expand further with each successive generation in a family, resulting in the phenomenon of clinical anticipation, with the age at onset tending to become younger with each generation.[28] The step-up in CTG repeat length tends to be greater for offspring of affected mothers than of affected fathers, hence explaining why the mother is invariably the affected parent in the congenital form.[29] The CTG expansion may exert influence on several genes in the vicinity of the DM protein kinase, as well as on this gene itself.[30]

Facioscapulohumeral muscular dystrophy. In FSHD, there is broad correlation between the size of the residual DNA fragment resulting from the 3.3 kb repeat deletion and the age at onset, with the earliest childhood onset cases (who may require a wheelchair by 20 years) having the smallest residual DNA fragment lengths.[31,32] Current opinion favours a putative gene whose normal expression in muscle is either regulated by the repeat sequences or, if located closely centromeric to these in the 4q35 chromosome region, affected adversely by their reduction in number. This could operate either through disturbance of the normal folding of DNA in this region or through heterochromatic inactivation spreading more proximally if the distance between the putative gene and the telomere is reduced by the deletion.[33] There is also some suggestion that clinical anticipation is observed in families but, since the deletion size remains constant in a family, such a phenomenon would currently be difficult to explain.[31,32,34] Very mild symptoms in the parent of a severe childhood onset case may be due to the mutation arising first in mitotic cell division in the parent, who will be a germinal and somatic mosaic for the mutation.[35,36] Parental mosaicism has been recorded from DNA study in at least 20% of otherwise clinically 'new mutation' cases of FSHD.[23]

Other muscular dystrophies. Although correlations between specific mutations and severity of phenotype will undoubtedly exist in other muscular dystrophies, the number of patients recognised with any particular mutation is only now becoming sufficient to enable such studies to be made.

Genetic management of families

The presence of a uniform mutation mechanism or the identification of the specific mutation(s) in a family enables accurate assessment of genetic risk, particularly for:

- carrier detection for X-linked dystrophies;
- presymptomatic detection or clarification of affected/unaffected status in dominant dystrophies; and
- accurate prenatal diagnosis in any dystrophy.

Without knowledge of the specific mutation, genetic management must rely on indirect DNA analysis using DNA polymorphisms from within or closely linked to the presumed disease gene. For carrier risk assessment in DMD, these indirect DNA results are combined with results of serum CK levels in the post-pubertal females at risk. For some families, this can still leave an unsatisfactory situation, as illustrated in the following genuine case history (see Fig 6).

Case history

A 36 year old married woman, whose elder brother had died at age 14 years from DMD, wished to commence a family. There was no known past family history of DMD, but her mother and maternal grandmother had both been only children. DNA samples were available from her normal brother and from both parents. CK levels of 153 iu/l and 126 iu/l in her mother and herself led to estimated carrier risks of 88% and 60% for her mother and herself, respectively. DNA polymorphic marker analysis from across the dystrophin gene was unhelpful in clarifying her carrier risk because she shared only the 3' half of her dystrophin gene with her

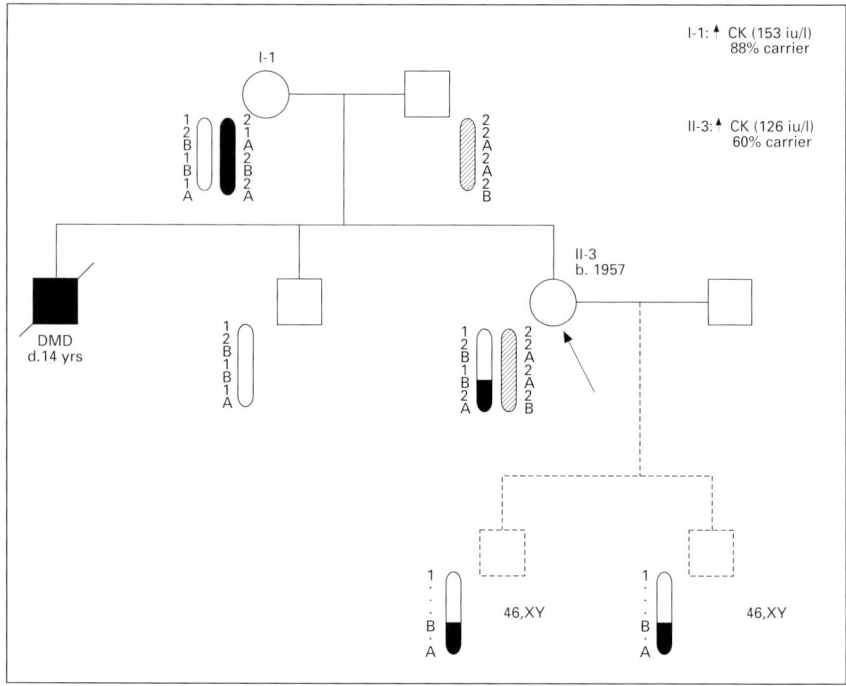

Fig 6. *Illustrative genuine family case history.* This shows the difficulties in one family of necessary reliance on indirect linked polymorphisms for Duchenne muscular dystrophy (DMD) genetic risk assessment, and highlights the need for the availability of efficient techniques for family-specific mutation detection. The DNA typing is illustrated for seven probes from across the dystrophin gene (5' end ... DYSII, Cf56B, STR45, Cf56A, STR49, MP1P, STRH1 ... 3' end) (CK = creatine kinase) (DNA typing by M Williams and L Tyfield, Southmead Hospital, Bristol).

normal brother due to a recombination event, the 5' half being from the opposite maternal copy which carries all the genetic risk.

She became pregnant, and from an 11-week chorion villus biopsy (CVB) the fetus was identified as male and carrying intact the high-risk copy of her DMD gene markers. Given an estimated 60% risk of DMD in the fetus, she elected for termination of pregnancy. No deletion was detected in the fetal DNA, thereby to some extent reducing her carrier risk. Following two failed attempts at *in vitro* fertilisation and pre-implantation sexing, the couple elected for a second pregnancy, and again for a CVB test. Although the result was exactly the same as in the first pregnancy, the couple did not feel they could terminate this pregnancy. Unfortunately, the baby boy proved to have inherited DMD with a very high infantile CK level (4,150 iu/l). In retrospect, it might have been wise to study dystrophin immunostaining on muscle tissue from the aborted fetus (if this could have been obtained), and possibly to have requested a muscle biopsy from the woman or her mother to test for variation in dystrophin immunostaining of individual muscle fibres – a feature in symptomatically manifesting carrier females as a consequence of X-inactivation.[37] The situation might have been avoided, however, if it had been possible to identify a specific dystrophin gene mutation in DNA from the woman or her mother.

Genetic management in Duchenne/Becker muscular dystrophy

Family-specific mutation detection

The choice of methods used to detect family-specific mutation in DMD/BMD, EDMD or LGMD depends on the expected relative frequency of different mutation types. Dystrophin mutations causing DMD/BMD occur as follows:[38,39]

- deletion of exons or part of exons: 65%,
- duplication of exons or part of exons: 7%,
- nonsense mutations introducing STOP codon and splice-site mutations: 10%,
- others (base substitutions, etc): 18%.

Deletions are detected most efficiently using a multiplex PCR technique.[20] Using DNA primers from each end of several different exons, the latter can be amplified simultaneously and all 78 exons covered by a small number of similar tests. Any exon involved in a deletion will fail to amplify, or give a shortened DNA fragment if the deletion is contained within that exon.

Duplications can also be detected from standardly extracted peripheral leukocyte DNA by a similar multiplex PCR technique, but with addition of a fluorescent marker to tag the DNA fragments, and hence be able to measure exon dosage from quantification of the fluorescence.[39] Alternatively, the use of PFGE to enable separation of very long DNA fragments following digestion by rare-cutting restriction enzymes will identify duplications as well as any 'junction fragments' which result from deletions.[40] Unfortunately, the extraction of DNA of sufficiently high quality (ie molecular weight) suitable for PFGE analysis requires that the blood sample be received fresh in the laboratory within a few hours of being taken, which limits the general accessibility of this technique.

Nonsense mutations and *splice-site mutations* produce an altered length protein product. This can be detected using the protein truncation test, whereby DNA is reverse transcribed from the patient's mRNA and used for *in vitro* transcription and translation to study the length of the encoded protein product.[41] Dystrophin mRNA is required, so the starting material for such testing should ideally be fresh muscle tissue, although a small quantity of ectopic mRNA transcript can be isolated from fresh lymphocytes.[42] The accessibility of this technique is therefore also limited by practical considerations. It may become possible to induce dystrophin mRNA production in skin fibroblast cultures by incorporating into them an active muscle gene promoter, MyoD.[38,43]

Other missense point mutations can be detected from DNA by one of several labour-intensive methods, which may be based on single-strand conformational polymorphism, denaturing gradient gel electrophoresis, mismatch hybridisation and chemical cleavage, or direct sequencing of each exon in turn following PCR amplification.[44] Currently, the availability of these methods is still largely limited to the context of a laboratory's research programme.

Carrier testing

Carrier risk can be estimated from the combination of pedigree structure, CK level and linked DNA marker analysis, as discussed above. If the dystrophin mutation in the family is known to be a deletion or duplication, carriers may be detected with certainty from quantitative fluorescent multiplex PCR (QFMPCR)[39] or PFGE analysis.[40] Some large deletions may also be detectable using fluorescent *in situ* hybridisation on to a chromosome spread.[45]

For known family-specific missense mutations, PCR primers could be constructed to provide a direct assay for presence or absence of the particular mutation. If no material is available from an affected male, the QFMPCR or PFGE methods, or a new Southern blot method which detects novel junction fragments,[46] can also be used to screen female relatives for evidence of carrying a deletion or duplication. Muscle biopsy with dystrophin immunostaining is probably helpful only for carrier detection where a woman is known to exhibit symptoms – then acting more as a diagnostic test.[1,37]

Other genetic aspects: mutation and mosaicism

Although one-third of apparently isolated cases of DMD arise from fresh, new mutation (the mother being a carrier in two-thirds),

15% of mothers with no evidence from blood for being carriers of the DMD mutation identified in their affected son are at risk of having a second affected child. These mothers have germline mosaicism for the mutation, whereby the original mutation event has occurred in a pre-oocyte mitotic cell division.[47] Therefore, a minimum 15% risk to any male infant who inherits the same maternal dystrophin gene markers as his brother with DMD must be discussed in genetic counselling for DMD.[44] A similar relative frequency of parental mutational mosaicism is also observed with apparently isolated cases of FSHD.[23,25]

Furthermore, it is now known that point mutations in the dystrophin gene arise predominantly during spermatogenesis, whereas deletions and duplications arise as mutations predominantly during oogenesis.[48] Therefore, the mother of a DMD/BMD boy who has a point mutation may have a greater than two-thirds chance of being a carrier, whereas the chance of a deletion or duplication being familial may be less than two-thirds. This emphasises the need to identify the family-specific mutation, since the ones hardest to identify may be those most likely to confer risk to the wider family.

This also seems to apply to fully affected females with DMD, in the majority of whom the DMD mutation is paternal in origin if it is due to skewed X-inactivation.[49] Other possible causes in fully affected females are:

- 45,XO karyotype,
- X-autosome translocation,
- skewed X-inactivation associated with monozygous twinning, and
- (rarely) homozygosity.

However, in any fully affected female, an alternative diagnosis of severe childhood LGMD should also be considered.

Prospects for treatment/gene therapy in Duchenne/Becker muscular dystrophy

To date, treatments in DMD are palliative and symptom-based, rather than corrective. These include physical therapy to prevent contractures and maintain posture (including use of standing frames), and spinal rod surgery. Various treatment trials have been carried out (eg with vitamin E), without any convincing benefit.[1] There is some evidence now from the USA that the use of steroids may delay onset of loss of ambulation, and multicentre UK trials are being considered.[1,50] Perhaps the single most effective therapy to date is the use of nocturnal ventilation when the boys are entering respiratory failure; preliminary indications are that this can convert an expected six-month survival from that time to a 75% six-year survival (A Symonds; personal communication, 1997).[51]

The concept of replacing part or all of a faulty DMD gene in muscle cells with a corrected version is enticing, but will be hampered both by the size of the dystrophin gene and by the difficulties of delivery of any potentially corrective DNA or cells to the target muscle tissue. Encouragement that a method of treatment may eventually be found can be taken from the natural occurrence of occasional revertant (dystrophin-expressing) muscle fibres in boys with DMD, as shown in Fig 4(d).[52,53] The availability of the *mdx* mouse, which has a mouse-dystrophin gene mutation,[54] provides an animal system in which any proposed somatic therapy can first be tested.

Treatment approaches

The methods tested so far have had little success, resulting at most in only a few dystrophin-producing muscle fibres for a relatively short period of time following each round of treatment.[55,56] These methods have included:

- Direct injection of dystrophin gene DNA or mRNA into muscle cells.[57]
- Vector-mediated gene (or exon) delivery, using adenovirus, retrovirus or liposomes.[55,58,59]
- Myoblast transfer, following *in vitro* recombinant DNA manipulation.[60–62]
- Fibroblast transfer, also containing recombinant DNA, and with MyoD to stimulate expression of muscle-specific genes, and in effect, differentiation into myoblasts.[63]
- Attempts to induce the skipping of faulty exons in the transcription or translation of dystrophin DNA/RNA.[52,53,56]
- Attempts to upregulate the expression of utrophin, a dystrophin-like protein encoded by a gene on chromosome 6q, which may be able to compensate for an absence of dystrophin.[64] This is perhaps the current potentially most promising approach.

Newborn screening programme

Population screening of newborn male infants for DMD is feasible by CK assay from the Guthrie blood spot at 10 days of age.[65] However, without clear treatment benefits (which an eventual successful form of gene replacement therapy could provide) it has been generally assumed that the distress caused to unsuspecting parents by predicting that a healthy neonate would develop DMD would preclude any genetic benefit that would accrue from being able to avoid families already having two affected sons by the time the elder boy is diagnosed by traditional methods. Initial results from an ongoing research study, based in the Institute of Medical Genetics in Cardiff[65] in fact suggest that, with voluntary entry into the newborn screening research programme, the parental distress is not as great as feared. It is probably exceeded in the unscreened population by the anxiety of those parents whose son's diagnosis of DMD fails to be recognised until many months or years after they first become concerned by his symptoms, and certainly by the distress of those who find, with traditional diagnosis, that they already have two affected children.[66]

Early diagnosis does not, however, seem able so far to lead to any additional intervention which can alter the prognosis for an affected boy himself. Until gene therapy becomes a reality, the medical benefit of newborn screening or, alternatively, of screening all non-walking males at 18 months of age, is only for the genetic aspects of care and a probable overall reduction in anxiety (AJ Clarke; personal communication, 1996).

References

1   Emery AEH. *Duchenne muscular dystrophy*, 2nd edn. Oxford Monographs on Medical Genetics No 24. Oxford: Oxford University Press, 1993.

2   Emery AEH (ed). *Diagnostic criteria for neuromuscular disorders*, 2nd edn. London: Royal Society of Medicine Press, 1997.

3   Bushby KMD. The limb-girdle muscular dystrophies. In: Emery AEH (ed). *Diagnostic criteria for neuromuscular disorders*, 2nd edn. London: Royal Society of Medicine Press, 1997: 17–22.

4   Dubowitz V. *Muscle disorders in childhood*, 2nd edn. London: Saunders, 1988.

5   Walton JN. *Disorders of voluntary muscle*, 5th edn. Edinburgh: Churchill Livingstone, 1988.

6   Jardine PE, Koch MC, Lunt PW, Maynard J, *et al.* De novo facioscapulohumeral muscular dystrophy defined by DNA probe p13E-11 (D4F104S1). *Archives of Disease in Childhood* 1994; **71**: 221–7.

7   Kaplan J-C, Fontaine B. Neuromuscular disorders: gene location. *Neuromuscular Disorders* 1997; **7**: I–XI.

8   Francke U, Ochs HD, de Martinville B, Giacalone J, *et al.* Minor Xp21 chromosome deletion in a male associated with expression of Duchenne muscular dystrophy, chronic granulomatous disease, retinitis pigmentosa, and McLeod syndrome. *American Journal of Human Genetics* 1985; **37**: 250–67.

9 Monaco AP, Neve RL, Colletti-Feener C, Bertelson CJ, *et al.* Isolation of candidate cDNAs for portions of the Duchenne muscular dystrophy gene. *Nature* 1986; **323**: 646–50.

10 Ahn AH, Kunkel LM. The structural and functional diversity of dystrophin. *Nature Genetics* 1993; **3**: 283–91.

11 Ervasti JM, Campbell KP. Membrane organization of the dystrophin-glycoprotein complex. *Cell* 1991; **66**: 1–20.

12 Vainzof M, Passos-Bueno MR, Canovas M. The sarcoglycan complex in the six autosomal recessive limb-girdle muscular dystrophies. *Human Molecular Genetics* 1996; **5**: 1963–9.

13 Roberds S, Leturcq F, Allamand V, Piccolo F, *et al.* Missense mutations in the adhalin gene linked to autosomal recessive muscular dystrophy. *Cell* 1994; **78**: 625–33.

14 Noguchi S, McNally EM, Ben Othmane K, Hagiwara Y, *et al.* Mutations in the dystrophin-associated protein γ-sarcoglycan in chromosome 13 muscular dystrophy. *Science* 1995; **270**: 819–22.

15 Nagano A, Koga R, Ogawa M, Kurano Y, *et al.* Emerin deficiency at the nuclear membrane in patients with Emery-Dreifuss muscular dystrophy. *Nature Genetics* 1996; **12**: 254–9.

16 Yates JRW. Workshop report. 43rd European Neuromuscular Centre international workshop on Emery-Dreifuss muscular dystrophy, 22 June 1996, Naarden, The Netherlands. *Neuromuscular Disorders* 1997; **7**: 67–9.

17 Helbling-Leclerc A, Zhang X, Topaloglu H, Cruaud C, *et al.* Mutations in the laminin alpha 2-chain gene (LAMA2) cause merosin-deficient congenital muscular dystrophy. *Nature Genetics* 1995; **11**: 216–8.

18 Richard I, Broux O, Allamand V, Fougerousse F, *et al.* Mutations in the proteolytic enzyme, calpain 3, cause limb-girdle muscular dystrophy type 2A. *Cell* 1995; **81**: 27–40.

19 Hodgson SV, Hart K, Abbs S, Heckmatt J, *et al.* Correlation of clinical and deletion data in Duchenne and Becker muscular dystrophy. *Journal of Medical Genetics* 1989; **26**: 682–3.

20 Beggs AH, Koenig M, Boyce FM, Kunkel LM. Detection of 98% of DMD/BMD gene deletions by polymerase chain reaction. *Human Genetics* 1990; **86**: 45–8.

21 van Deutekom JC, Wijmenga C, van Tienhoven EA, Gruter AM, *et al.* FSHD associated DNA rearrangements are due to deletions of integral copies of a 3.2 kb tandemly repeated unit. *Human Molecular Genetics* 1993; **2**: 2037–42.

22 van Deutekom JCT, Bakker E, Lemmers RJLF, van der Wielen MJR, *et al.* Evidence for subtelomeric exchange of 3.3 kb tandemly repeated units between chromosomes 4q35 and 10q26: implications for genetic counselling and etiology of FSHD1. *Human Molecular Genetics* 1996; **5**: 1997–2003.

23 Lunt PW. Workshop Report. 44th International Workshop on Facioscapulohumeral Muscular Dystrophy: Molecular Studies, 19–21 July 1996, Naarden, The Netherlands. *Neuromuscular Disorders* 1998; **8**: 126–30.

24 Harley HG, Rundle SA, MacMillan JC, Myring J, *et al.* Size of the

unstable CTG repeat sequence in relation to phenotype and parental transmission in myotonic dystrophy. *American Journal of Human Genetics* 1993; **52**: 1164–74.

25   Nicholson LVB, Johnson MA, Gardner-Medwin D, Bhattacharya S, *et al.* Heterogeneity of dystrophin expression in patients with Duchenne and Becker muscular dystrophy. *Acta Neuropathologica (Berlin)* 1990; **80**: 239–50.

26   Koenig M, Beggs AH, Moyer M, Scherpf S, *et al.* The molecular basis for Duchenne versus Becker muscular dystrophy: correlation of severity with type of deletion. *American Journal of Human Genetics* 1989; **45**: 498–506.

27   Rapaport D, Passos-Bueno MR, Brandao L, Love D, *et al.* Apparent association of mental retardation and specific patterns of deletions screened with probes Cf56a and Cf23a in Duchenne muscular dystrophy. *American Journal of Medical Genetics* 1991; **39**: 437–41.

28   Harper PS, Harley HG, Reardon W, Shaw DJ. Anticipation in myotonic dystrophy – new light on an old problem. *American Journal of Human Genetics* 1992; **51**: 10–6.

29   Lavedan C, Hofmann-Radvanyi H, Shelbourne P, Rabes JP, *et al.* Myotonic dystrophy: size- and sex-dependent dynamics of CTG meiotic instability, and somatic mosaicism. *American Journal of Human Genetics* 1993; **52**: 875–83.

30   Harris S, Moncrieff C, Johnson K. Myotonic dystrophy: will the real gene please step forward! Review. *Human Molecular Genetics* 1996; **5**: 1417–23.

31   Lunt PW, Jardine PE, Koch MC, Maynard J, *et al.* Correlation between fragment size at D4F104S1 and age at onset or at wheelchair use, with a possible generational effect, accounts for much phenotypic variation in 4q35-facioscapulohumeral muscular dystrophy (FSHD). *Human Molecular Genetics* 1995; **4**: 951–8 (erratum: 1243–4).

32   Tawil R, Forrester J, Griggs RC, Mendell J, *et al.* Evidence for anticipation and association of deletion size with severity in facioscapulohumeral muscular dystrophy. *Annals of Neurology* 1996; **39**: 744–8.

33   Winokur ST, Bengtsson U, Feddersen J, Matthews KD, *et al.* The DNA rearrangement associated with facioscapulohumeral muscular dystrophy involves a heterochromatin associated repetitive element: implications for a role of chromatin structure in the pathogenesis of the disease. *Chromosome Research* 1994; **2**: 225–34.

34   Zatz M, Marie SK, Passos-Bueno MR, Vainzof M, *et al.* High proportion of new mutations and possible anticipation in Brazilian facioscapulohumeral muscular dystrophy families. *American Journal of Human Genetics* 1995; **56**: 99–105.

35   Kohler J, Rupilius B, Otto M, Bathke K, Koch MC. Germ-Line mosaicism in 4q35 facioscapulohumeral muscular dystrophy (FSHD1A) occurring predominantly in oogenesis. *Human Genetics* 1996; **98**: 485–90.

36   Upadhyaya M, Maynard J, Osborn M, Jardine P, *et al.* Germinal mosaicism in facioscapulohumeral muscular dystrophy (FSHD). *Muscle and Nerve* 1995; Suppl 2: S45–9.

37   Clerk A, Rodillo E, Heckmatt JZ, Dubowitz V, *et al.* Characterisation of

dystrophin in carriers of Duchenne muscular dystrophy. *Journal of Neurological Science* 1991; **102**: 197–205.

38   Roest PAM, Bout M, van der Tuijn AC, Ginjaar IB, *et al.* Splicing mutations in DMD/BMD detected by RT-PCR/PTT: detection of a 19AA insertion in the cysteine rich domain of dystrophin compatible with BMD. *Journal of Medical Genetics* 1996; **33**: 935–9.

39   Yau SC, Bobrow M, Mathew CG, Abbs SJ. Accurate diagnosis of carriers of deletions and duplications in Duchenne/Becker muscular dystrophy by fluorescent dosage analysis. *Journal of Medical Genetics* 1996; **33**: 550–8.

40   den Dunnen JT, Bakker E, Klein Breteler EG, Pearson PL, *et al.* Direct detection of more than 50% of the Duchenne muscular dystrophy mutations by field inversion gels. *Nature* 1987; **329**: 640–2.

41   Roest PAM, Roberts RG, Sugino S, van Ommen GJB, den Dunnen JT. Protein truncation test (PTT) for rapid detection of translation-termination mutations. *Human Molecular Genetics* 1993; **2**: 1719–21.

42   Roberts RG, Barby TFM, Manners E, Bobrow M, Bentley DR. Direction detection of dystrophin gene rearrangements by analysis of dystrophin mRNA in peripheral blood lymphocytes. *American Journal of Human Genetics* 1991; **49**: 298–310.

43   Roest PAM, van der Tuijn AC, Ginjaar HB, Hoeben RC, *et al.* Application of in vitro myo-differentiation of non-muscle cells to enhance gene expression and facilitate analysis of muscle proteins. *Neuromuscular Disorders* 1996; **6**: 195–202.

44   van Essen AJ, Kneppers ALJ, van der Hout AH, Scheffer H, *et al.* The clinical and molecular genetic approach to Duchenne and Becker muscular dystrophy: an updated protocol. *Journal of Medical Genetics* 1997; **34**: 805–12.

45   Ried T, Mahler V, Vogt P, Blonden L, *et al.* Direct carrier detection by in situ suppression hybridization with cosmid clones of the Duchenne/Becker muscular dystrophy locus *Human Genetics* 1990; **85**: 581–6.

46   Yamagishi H, Kato S, Hiraishi Y, Ishihara T, *et al.* Identification of carriers of Duchenne/Becker muscular dystrophy by a novel method based on detection of junction fragments in the dystrophin gene. *Journal of Medical Genetics* 1996; **33**: 1027–31.

47   Passos-Bueno MR, Bakker E, Kneppers AL, Takata RI, *et al.* Different mosaicism frequencies for proximal and distal DMD mutations indi-cate difference in etiology and recurrence risk. *American Journal of Human Genetics* 1992; **51**: 1150–5.

48   Grimm T, Meng G, Liechti-Gallati S, Bettecken I, *et al.* On the origin of deletions and point mutations in Duchenne muscular dystrophy: most deletions arise in oogenesis and most point mutations result from events in spermatogenesis. *Journal of Medical Genetics* 1994; **31**: 183–6.

49   Pegoraro E, Schimke RN, Arahata K, Hayashi Y, *et al.* Detection of new paternal dystrophin gene mutations in isolated cases of dystrophinopathy in females. *American Journal of Human Genetics* 1994; **54**: 989–1003.

50   Angelini C. Therapeutic trial in DMD: past research and future trends. *Muscle and Nerve* 1994; Suppl 1: S66/W-27-1.

51 Rutgers MR Workshop Report. 39th European Neuromuscular Centre International Workshop on Respiratory Insufficiency and Ventilatory Support, 26–28 January 1996, Naarden, The Netherlands. *Neuromuscular Disorders* 1996; **6**: 431–5.

52 Nicholson LVB. The 'rescue' of dystrophin synthesis in boys with Duchenne muscular dystrophy. *Neuromuscular Disorders* 1993; **3**: 525–31.

53 Thanh LT, Nguyen TM, Helliwell TR, Morris GE. Characterisation of revertant muscle fibers in Duchenne muscular dystrophy, using exon-specific monoclonal antibodies against dystrophin. *American Journal of Human Genetics* 1995; **56**: 725–31.

54 Sicinski P, Geng Y, Ryder-Cook AS, Barnard EA, *et al.* The molecular basis of muscular dystrophy in the mdx mouse: a point mutation. *Science* 1989; **244**: 1578–80.

55 Kumar-Singh R, Chamberlain JS. Encapsulated adenovirus mini-chromosomes allow delivery and expression of a 14 kb dystrophin cDNA to muscle cells. *Human Molecular Genetics* 1996; **5**: 913–21.

56 Bakker E. Duchenne and Becker muscular dystrophy (D/BMD): diagnosis, gene defect, genotype phenotype correlation, is gene therapy next? *Abstract of presentation at European Neuromuscular Centre Symposium on Recent Advances and Future Prospects in Neuromuscular Disorders*, 23–25 May 1997, Naarden, The Netherlands.

57 Acsadi G, Dickson G, Love DR, Jani A, *et al.* Human dystrophin expression in mdx mice after intramuscular injection of DNA constructs. *Nature* 1991; **352**: 815–8.

58 Ragot T, Vincent N, Chafey P. Efficient adenovirus-mediated transfer of a human minidystrophin gene to skeletal muscle of mdx mice. *Nature* 1993; **361**: 647–50.

59 Dunkley MG, Wells DJ, Walsh FS, Dickson G. Direct retroviral-mediated transfer of a dystrophin minigene into mdx mouse muscle in vivo. *Human Molecular Genetics* 1993; **2**: 717–23.

60 Partridge TA, Morgan JE, Coulton GR, Hoffman EP, *et al.* Conversion of mdx myofibres from dystrophin-negative to -positive by injection of normal myoblasts. *Nature* 1989; **337**: 176–9.

61 Mendell JR, Kissel JT, Amato AA, King W, *et al.* Myoblast transfer in the treatment of Duchenne's muscular dystrophy. *New England Journal of Medicine* 1995; **333**: 832–8.

62 Partridge TA, Davies KE. Myoblast-based gene therapies. In: Lever AML, Goodfellow P (eds). *Gene therapy*. Edinburgh: Churchill Livingstone; *British Medical Bulletin* 1995; **51**: 123–37.

63 Salvatori G, Ferrari G, Lattanzi L, Coletta M, *et al.* Ex vivo gene therapy for myopathies: how to get enough myogenic cells. In: Symposium on recent advances in diagnosis and therapy of neuromuscular diseases, Prato, Italy. *Neuromuscular disorders* 1996; **6**: S23/G1S3.

64 Tinsley JM, Potter AC, Phelps SR, Fisher R, *et al.* Amelioration of the dystrophic phenotype of mdx mice using a truncated utrophin transgene. *Nature* 1996; **384**: 349–53.

65 Bradley DM, Parsons EP, Clarke AJ. Experience with screening newborns for Duchenne muscular dystrophy in Wales. *British Medical Journal* 1993; **306**: 357–60.

66 Bowman JE. Screening newborn infants for Duchenne muscular dystrophy. *British Medical Journal* 1993; **306**: 349.

7 | Sex determination

J Ross Hawkins
Department of Paediatrics, University of Cambridge

Human genetic analysis need not be limited to classical single gene diseases but can be applied to any phenotype with a genetic component. In this chapter, the genetic analysis of patients with disorders of gonadal and sexual development is described. Several genes involved in sex determination have been identified. By studying how these genes interact, it should eventually be possible to understand the complex genetic pathway underlying this developmental mechanism.

Sexual development

Development of the sexual phenotype can be divided into three stages:

- gonadal sex determination;
- gonadal differentiation; and
- sexual differentiation.

The determination of gonadal sex is normally a direct consequence of the sex chromosome constitution: that is, 46,XX or 46,XY. The sex chromosome constitution is established at fertilisation, but it is believed that it is not until at about six weeks' gestation (just before the indifferent gonads begin to differentiate) that it instructs the path of gonadal development. This decision to proceed with either ovarian or testicular development is followed by the differentiation of the gonads into ovaries in XX individuals and testes in XY individuals. Sexual differentiation (the differentiation of the internal and external genitalia as female or male) follows from gonadal differentiation and occurs as a response to hormones produced by the differentiated gonads.

Biology of sex determination

Much of our knowledge of gonadal differentiation and sexual endocrinology stems from a series of experiments conducted by Jost over several decades.[1] He demonstrated that the presence or absence of testes causes male or female sexual development, respectively. Later, the specific testicular hormones were discovered:

- *Anti-Müllerian hormone*, secreted from the Sertoli cells, which causes the regression of the female internal genitalia.
- *Testosterone*, secreted from the Leydig cells, which maintains the development of the male internal genitalia.
- The testosterone derivative, *dihydrotestosterone*, which stimulates the development of the male external genitalia.

There are many opportunities for errors with all the complex developmental systems but, unlike most of them, defects in sexual development are not expected to be lethal but to cause the sex of the individual to be at odds with the sex chromosome constitution. Studies of human individuals with XX and XY sex reversal have been fundamental to our understanding of the molecular processes underlying testis determination and the early steps of gonadal differentiation.

Cloning the testis determining factor

The findings in the late 1950s that Turner and Klinefelter syndrome patients have 45,X and 47,XXY karyotypes, respectively,[2,3] gave the first indication that the Y chromosome is a dominant inducer of male development. The gene or genes responsible for this activity became known as the testis determining factor (*TDF*). It was believed that it would be possible to use the information derived by cloning *TDF* as a key into the pathway of testis determination, thus facilitating the identification and characterisation of the other genes involved.

It was suggested by Ferguson-Smith in 1966[1] that aberrant recombination between the X and Y chromosomes at meiosis could cause loss of *TDF* from the Y chromosome and gain of *TDF* on the X, to result in XY female and XX male development, respectively (Fig 1). Since then, most human genetic studies of sex determination have focused upon these individuals. Molecular studies mapped the position of *TDF* immediately proximal to the 'pseudoautosomal' X-Y pairing region on the short arm of the

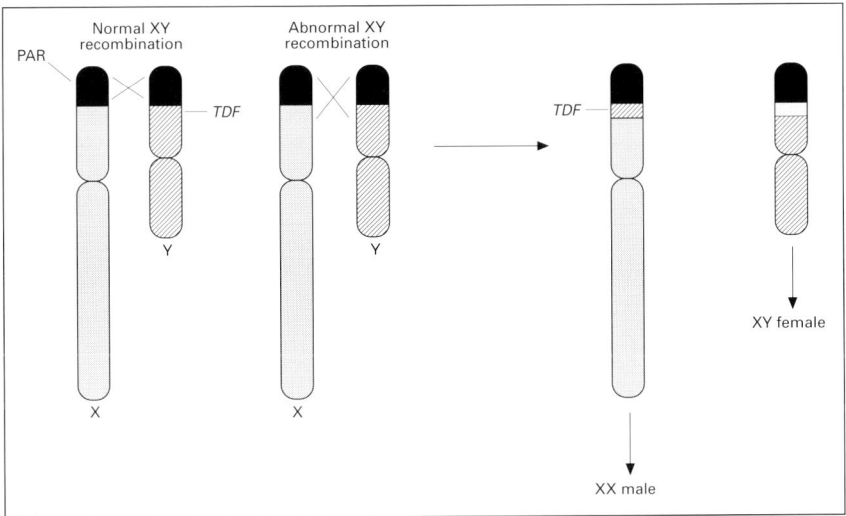

Fig 1. *Aberrant X-Y recombination.* In male meiosis, a recombination event occurs between the pseudoautosomal regions (PAR) of the X and Y chromosomes. In rare instances, X-specific and Y-specific DNA sequences are exchanged. If this includes the testis determining factor (TDF), the gametes derived generate XX males and XY females.

Y chromosome. The cloning and analysis of this region revealed one gene which was named *SRY* (sex determining region of the Y gene).[5]

The *SRY* gene

Expression studies of the mouse homologue of *SRY* (*Sry*) showed that in the embryo the gene is expressed in the somatic cells of the genital ridge for only about 36 hours immediately prior to the onset of overt testicular differentiation.[6] DNA sequence analysis of *SRY* predicted SRY protein to be just 204 amino acids in length and to contain only one recognisable domain. This domain, known as the 'HMG-box', is a DNA-binding motif, first observed in the high mobility group (HMG) chromatin structural proteins. Proof that *SRY* was indeed *TDF* came from the identification of mutations in the *SRY* gene of *SRY*-positive XY females[7] and the production of chromosomally female mice transgenic for *Sry* which developed as males.[8] The latter experiment also indicated that *SRY* is the sole component of *TDF*, and that no other genes on the Y chromosome are necessary for testis development.

SRY mutations

To date, about 25 mutations in *SRY* have been published.[9] All but two are located in the HMG-box region, indicating that this is the major functional domain of the SRY protein. All the mutations were found in patients with complete XY gonadal dysgenesis, in whom there is a total failure of testis development due to the absence of a testis-determining signal.[10] These patients are sterile, so mutations cannot be inherited and must arise only as new mutations. Three of the described *SRY* mutations, however, defy this logic; in these cases, the mutations exist silently in carrier fathers. It is unclear so far why some mutations show variable penetrance whilst most do not. Only about 20% of XY complete gonadal dysgenesis patients have mutations in *SRY*, stressing that *SRY* does not act alone in testis determination and that a pathway of genes is likely to be required.

SRY biochemistry

Using a polymerase chain reaction-based selective amplification process, the sequence A/TAACAAT was identified as an *in vitro* consensus DNA binding sequence for SRY protein.[11] DNA binding studies on recombinant wild type and mutant SRY protein with labelled DNA containing the binding site demonstrated that SRY protein bends the DNA to which it binds.[12] Furthermore, a reduction in either the binding affinity or the bend angle results in gonadal dysgenesis.[13] Interestingly, the reduction of the binding and bending activities of the inherited *SRY* mutations is less severe than for the *de novo* mutations. It is therefore likely that SRY acts as a transcription factor by bringing together other linearly spaced bound factors, facilitating their interaction.

SOX genes

When *SRY* was first used as a probe on Southern blots it was noticed that the resulting autoradiographic image had a high background, with many faint additional bands.[5] It was soon realised that these bands represented a family of related genes with similar HMG-box regions. These genes have been named *SOX* genes (<u>S</u>RY-related HMG-b<u>ox</u>), and defined as having 60% or more amino acid similarity to the SRY HMG-box. About 20 *SOX* genes have been identified in humans and mice, of which only a handful have been well characterised. They are all expressed in the embryo and/or gametes, and appear to be involved in diverse embryonic processes such as neuronal and skeletal development.

SOX9 and campomelic dysplasia

Campomelic dysplasia (CD) is a rare congenital disorder of skeletal development, frequently associated with complete or partial XY sex reversal.[14] The abnormality of sexual development stems from abnormal gonadal development rather than a defect of gonadal function. The gonadal defects (complete and partial gonadal dysgenesis) are observed only in XY patients, indicating a defect in testis determination rather than a generalised defect of gonadal development.

Balanced chromosomal translocations involving chromosome 17q were found in several cases of CD, indicating the location of the gene(s) responsible for the disorder.[15] Following DNA cloning studies, the break-points were found to lie close to the *SOX9* gene.[16] Mutation analysis of *SOX9* in non-translocation CD cases identified heterozygous mutations distributed throughout the entire gene. These mutations were found in both XX female and XY female CD patients, showing that disruption of *SOX9* is responsible for both the CD and the sex reversal phenotypes.

Expression of SOX9

Expression studies of *SOX9* indicated how this gene might cause these two diverse phenotypes when mutated. *SOX9* has two main sites of expression in the embryo:

The sites of chondrogenesis. In chondrocytes, SOX9 protein has been shown to be a potent activator of the type II collagen gene. It is therefore likely that a reduction in the level of SOX9 protein leads to a reduction in the levels of collagen II, and subsequently (indirectly) to a reduction in other cartilage matrix proteins, leading to skeletal malformation.[17,18]

The developing gonad. In the developing gonad, *SOX9* shows differential expression after the period of *SRY* expression. Expression is maintained throughout testis differentiation, but is extinguished in the developing ovary.[19] This is therefore highly suggestive that *SOX9* plays a key role in testis development.

SOX9 mutations

Over 20 mutations in *SOX9* have been found in CD patients.[9] Unlike *SRY*, the mutations are not concentrated in the HMG-box region but distributed throughout the gene. Analysis of the mutation type, position and resulting phenotype has failed to find a correlation between genotype and phenotype.[20] This is demonstrated well by identical mutations found in an XY male patient and an XY female patient. Despite the paucity of understanding of how genotype leads to phenotype, it is clear from the expression and mutation studies that *SOX9* has independent functions in skeletal and gonadal development.

SOX9 and sex reversal

Given that *SOX9* is likely to have an important role in testis development, it might be expected that some *SOX9* mutations could result in sex reversal in the absence of CD, but mutation screening of DNA samples from nearly 50 XY female patients has not detected any *SOX9* mutations.[20,21] These findings support the hypothesis that there are no discrete functional domains for the testis and bone developmental properties of *SOX9*, and that the sex reversal phenotype associated with CD shows variable penetrance.

Wilms tumour gene and gonadal development

The Wilms tumour gene (*WT1*), originally isolated as an oncogene involved in the aetiology of the childhood kidney cancer, Wilms tumour, has been shown to be expressed in the developing genital ridge from its earliest stages. Mutations in *WT1* can result in the Denys-Drash syndrome (DDS), which features renal failure together with gonadal and genital abnormalities.[22] The gonadal anomalies associated with DDS are not found only in XY patients, indicating that *WT1* has no, or little, role in the sexual differentiation of the gonads. Mice lacking the WT1 protein suffer failure of kidney and gonadal development.[23] Taken together, these data indicate that *WT1* is necessary for the commitment and maintenance of gonadal tissue.

FTZ-F1 and gonadal differentiation

The orphan nuclear receptor steroidogenic factor 1 (SF1) is a key regulator of enzymes involved in steroid production, including the sex hormones.[24] The gene encoding SF1, known as *FTZ-F1*, is expressed in all primary steroidogenic tissues, including the testes and ovaries. In addition to a well established role in the regulation of steroid production, however, SF1 has been heavily implicated in the development and differentiation of the gonads because:

- the expression profile of *FTZ-F1* in the gonads is similar to that of *SOX9*; and
- *FTZ-F1* null mice suffer the loss of both adrenal and gonadal structures.[24,25]

The exact role of SF1 in the developing gonad is far from clear, but it appears to be necessary for the maintenance of the gonadal tissue as well as being involved in early testicular function.

DAX1 and dosage-dependent XY sex reversal

Another gene implicated in sex determination is the X-linked, adrenal hypoplasia congenita (AHC) gene, *DAX1*. Although structural mutations result in AHC, chromosomal rearrangements which cause duplication of the gene result in XY sex reversal.[26,27] Interestingly, *DAX1* expression in gonadal differentiation mirrors that of *SOX9* and *FTZ-F1*, in that it is specifically expressed in the developing ovary, suggesting that *DAX1* is an ovarian determinant or an inhibitor of testis determination.[28] However, despite its probable key role in sex determination, *DAX1* duplications appear to account for only a very small proportion of cases of XY sex reversal.

Other genes in gonadal differentiation

Cytogenetically visible deletions in patients with XX or XY gonadal dysgenesis or with complete or partial sex reversal involving chromosome regions 9p, 10q and 18p implicate other, as yet uncloned, genes. The 9p gene would appear to be the most significant of these putative gonadal differentiation genes. Deletions of the terminal region of 9p have been found in several patients with complete or partial sex reversal.[29] The patients with smaller deletions do not have other anomalies, suggesting that this gene is specifically expressed in the gonads. In addition to these genes in the human, strong linkage has been detected in the mouse to two loci and weak linkage to a third locus which influence the phenotype in Y-linked complete and partial sex reversal.[30] The cloning of these genes from both human and mouse is therefore eagerly awaited.

Summary

The characterisation of genetic abnormalities resulting in abnormal gonadal development has led to the mapping and cloning of several genes. Investigating their functions should lead to an understanding of the mechanisms of sex determination and gonadal differentiation. It has been established that the genes *WT1* and *FTZ-F1* are required for the maintenance of the gonadal tissue, with the latter having further roles in the differentiation and functions of the gonads. *SRY* is the trigger required for testis determination to take place, with *SOX9* probably acting closely downstream. *DAX1* appears to be an ovarian determinant, and perhaps an antagonist of *SRY*.

It is thus clear that we can already begin to assemble the pathway of genes which direct the processes of gonadal sex determination and differentiation (Fig 2).

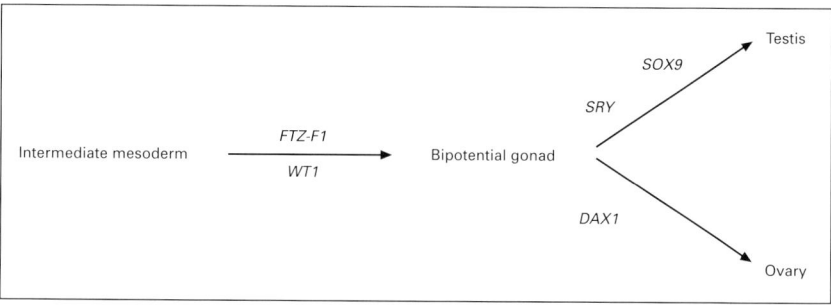

Fig 2. *Molecular events in early gonadal development.* The genes *WT1* and *FTZ-F1* are required for the formation and maintenance of the bipotential gonad from the intermediate mesoderm. *SRY* and *SOX9* are required for testis differentiation, and *DAX1* is probably necessary for ovarian differentiation.

References

1 Jost A, Vigier B, Prepin J, Perchellet JP. Studies on sex differentiation in mammals. *Recent Progress in Hormone Research* 1973; **29**: 1–41.

2 Ford CE, Jones KW, Polani P, De Almeida JC, Brigg JH. A sex chromosome abnormality in a case of gonadal sex dysgenesis (Turner's syndrome). *Lancet* 1959; **i**: 711–3.

3 Jacobs PA, Strong JA. A case of human intersexuality having a possible XXY sex determining mechanism. *Nature* 1959; **183**: 302–3.

4 Ferguson-Smith MA. X-Y chromosomal interchange in the aetiology of true hermaphroditism and XX Klinefelter's syndrome. *Lancet* 1966; **ii**: 475–6.

5   Sinclair AH, Berta P, Palmer MS, Hawkins JR, *et al.* A gene from the human sex-determining region encodes a protein with homology to a conserved DNA-binding motif. *Nature* 1990; **346**: 240–4.

6   Koopman P, Munsterberg A, Capel B, Vivian N, Lovell-Badge R. Expression of a candidate sex-determining gene during mouse testis differentiation. *Nature* 1990; **348**: 450–2.

7   Berta P, Hawkins JR, Sinclair AH, Taylor A, *et al.* Genetic evidence equating SRY and the testis determining factor. *Nature* 1990; **348**: 448–50.

8   Koopman P, Gubbay J, Vivian N, Goodfellow P, Lovell-Badge R. Male development of chromosomally female mice transgenic for *Sry*. *Nature* 1991; **351**: 117–21.

9   Cameron FJ, Sinclair AH. Mutations in SRY and SOX9: testis-determining genes. *Human Mutation* 1997; **9**: 388–95.

10 Berkovitz GD, Fechner PY, Zacur HW, Rock JA, *et al.* Clinical and pathologic spectrum of 46,XY gonadal dysgenesis: its relevance to the understanding of sex differentiation. *Medicine* 1991; **70**: 375–83.

11 Harley VR, Lovell-Badge R, Goodfellow PN. Definition of a consensus DNA, binding site for SRY. *Nucleic Acid Research* 1994; **22**: 1500–1.

12 Ferrari S, Harley VR, Pontiggia A, Goodfellow PN, Lovell-Badge R. SRY, like HMG1, recognizes sharp angles in DNA. *EMBO Journal* 1992; **11**: 4497–506.

13 Pontiggia A, Rimini R, Harley VR, Goodfellow PN, *et al.* Sex-reversing mutations affect the architecture of SRY-DNA complexes. *EMBO Journal* 1994; **13**: 6115–24.

14 Hovmoller ML, Osuna A, Eklof O, Fredge K, *et al.* Campomelic dwarfism. A genetically determined mesenchymal disorder combined with sex reversal. *Hereditas* 1977; **86**: 51–62.

15 Tommerup N, Schempp W, Meinecke P, Pedersen S, *et al.* Assignment of an autosomal sex reversal locus (SRA1) and campomelic dysplasia (CMPD1) to 17q24.3-q25.1. *Nature Genetics* 1993; **4**: 170–4.

16 Foster JW, Dominguez-Steglich MA, Guioli S, Kowk O, *et al.* Campomelic dysplasia and autosomal sex reversal caused by mutations in an SRY-related gene. *Nature* 1994; **372**: 525–30.

17 Wright E, Hargrave MR, Christiansen J, Cooper L, *et al.* The Sry-related gene Sox9 is expressed during chondrogenesis in mouse embryos. *Nature Genetics* 1995; **9**: 15–20.

18 Lefebvre V, Huang W, Harley VR, Goodfellow PN, de Crombrugghe B. SOX9 is a potent activator of the chondrocyte-specific enhancer of the pro alpha 1(II) collagen gene. *Molecular and Cellular Biology* 1997; **17**: 2336–46.

19 Morais da Silva S, Hacker A, Harley V, Goodfellow PN, *et al.* Sox9 expression during gonadal development implies a conserved role for the gene in testis differentiation in mammals and birds. *Nature Genetics* 1996; **14**: 62–8.

20 Meyer J, Sudbeck P, Held M, Wagner T, *et al.* Mutational analysis of the SOX9 gene in campomelic dysplasia and autosomal sex reversal – lack of genotype/phenotype correlations. *Human Molecular Genetics* 1997; **6**: 91–8.

21 Kwok C, Goodfellow PN, Hawkins JR. Evidence to exclude SOX9 as a

candidate gene for XY sex reversal without skeletal malformation. *Journal of Medical Genetics* 1996; **33**: 800–1.

22 Little M, Wells C. A clinical overview of WT1 gene-mutations. *Human Mutation* 1997; **9**: 209–25.

23 Kreidberg JA, Sariola H, Loring JM, Maeda M, *et al.* WT-1 is required for early kidney development. *Cell* 1993; **74**: 679–91.

24 Ikeda Y, Shen WH, Ingraham HA, Parker KL. Developmental expression of mouse steroidogenic factor-1, an essential regulator of the steroid hydroxylases. *Molecular Endocrinology* 1994; **8**: 654–62.

25 Luo XR, Ikeda YY, Parker KL. A cell-specific nuclear receptor is essential for adrenal and gonadal development and sexual-differentiation. *Cell* 1994; **77**: 481–90.

26 Zanaria E, Muscatelli F, Bardoni B, Strom TM, *et al.* An unusual member of the nuclear hormone-receptor superfamily responsible for X-linked adrenal hypoplasia congenita. *Nature* 1994; **372**: 635–41.

27 Bardoni B, Zanaria E, Guioli S, Floridia G, *et al.* A dosage sensitive locus at chromosome Xp21 is involved in male to female sex reversal. *Nature Genetics* 1994; **7**: 497–501.

28 Swain A, Zanaria E, Hacker A, Lovell-Badge R, Camerino G, *et al.* Mouse Dax1 expression is consistent with a role in sex determination as well as in adrenal and hypothalamus function. *Nature Genetics* 1996; **12**: 404–9.

29 Bennett CP, Docherty Z, Robb SA, Ramani P, *et al.* Deletion 9p and sex reversal. *Journal of Medical Genetics* 1993; **30**: 518–20.

30 Eicher EM, Washburn LL, Schork NJ, Lee BK, *et al.* Sex-determining genes on mouse autosomes identified by linkage analysis of C57BL/6J-YPOS sex reversal. *Nature Genetics* 1996; **14**: 206–9.

8 | Craniofacial disorders

Andrew Wilkie
*Institute of Molecular Medicine, John Radcliffe Hospital, Oxford,
and The Churchill and Oxford Craniofacial Unit, Radcliffe
Infirmary, Oxford*

The human skull is an exquisitely sculpted structure comprising 22 separate bones as well as 20 deciduous and 32 permanent teeth. Given this complexity, it is truly remarkable that the complex process of skull development is perfectly accomplished in the great majority of live born infants. Nevertheless, about one in 200 babies is born with craniofacial malformations,[1] which at the severe end of the spectrum can have devastating physical and psychological consequences (Fig 1). This chapter will focus on some of the major advances, mostly achieved within the past five years, in the identification of disease genes in human craniofacial malformation.

General principles

The following general principles relating to craniofacial malformations are emphasised:

1   Different malformations affect different aspects of craniofacial growth and arise at different times. A grasp of embryology is essential to interpret these abnormal mechanisms.

2   It is obviously difficult or impossible to study the processes of craniofacial malformation in human pregnancy. Animal (usually mouse) models are required. Much has been learnt from studying the effects of teratogens (notably ethanol, retinoids and phenytoin). More recently, it has become fairly routine to target precise mutations into the mouse genome, yielding a wealth of new genetic models.

3   Many genes involved in human craniofacial development have been shown to be the evolutionary counterparts (orthologues) of genes originally identified in the fruit-fly *Drosophila*. There may sometimes even be conservation of complete molecular

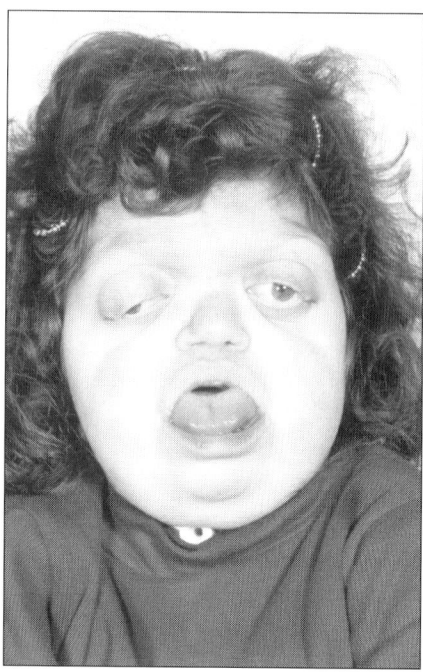

Fig 1. *Craniofacial appearance of a five year old girl with severe Pfeiffer syndrome.* She has craniosynostosis associated with raised intracranial pressure, choanal atresia and airway compromise requiring permanent tracheostomy and jejunostomy. She has required over 30 general anaesthetics, has severe learning difficulties, and needs 24-hour domiciliary care. Her condition is the consequence of a single heterozygous nucleotide substitution (G→T) in the fibroblast growth factor receptor 2 (*FGFR2*) gene.

pathways between these species (not necessarily in the same developmental context). This constitutes a triumphant vindication of the medical relevance of the genetic study of model organisms.

4   The study of malformation is a two-way process, in that the identification of disease genes provides new insights into normal mechanisms of development.

This chapter will discuss single gene disorders leading to skull malformation selected from the list in Table 1. It is intended to be illustrative rather than encyclopaedic – in any case, research advances so rapidly that the latter is an unrealistic goal. A more complete listing of single gene disorders associated with subtle facial dysmorphic features is provided by Winter.[20] For clinical descriptions of these disorders, the book by Gorlin and colleagues[21] is recommended.

Embryological considerations

The skull develops from two embryologically distinct tissues:

- the neural crest, which forms the facial skeleton, and
- the paraxial mesoderm, which forms the skull vault.

Surprisingly, the precise line of demarcation is still disputed.[22,23]
Normal human embryonic development is summarised in Fig 2.

Table 1. Some important disease genes in craniofacial disorders
(categorised by embryological mechanism, with those arising earliest at
the top). All are dominantly inherited, although the X-linked form of
Opitz G syndrome shows more severe features in males than females.

Gene	Location	Disorder	Suggested embryological mechanism	Ref
SHH	7q36	Holoprosencephaly	Midline deficiency of neural plate	2–6
GLI3	7p13	Greig cephalopolysyndactyly	Overgrowth of facial mesenchyme	7,8
MID1	Xp22	Opitz G syndrome	Abnormal midline patterning	9
PAX3	2q35	Waardenburg syndrome type 1	Defective neural crest migration	10
TCOF1	5q31–q33	Treacher Collins syndrome	1st and 2nd branchial arch deficiency	11,12
EYA1	8q13.3	Branchio-oto-renal syndrome	Incomplete obliteration of branchial cleft	13
COL2A1	12q13.11–q13.2	} Stickler syndrome	Incomplete fusion/ deficiency of palatal shelves	14
COL11A1	1p21			15
COL11A2	6p21.3			14
OSF2/CBFA1	6p21	Cleidocranial dysplasia	Failure to develop membrane bones	16
MSX2	5q34–35	Boston craniosynostosis	} Premature fusion of cranial sutures	17
FGFR1	8p11.2–p12	Pfeiffer syndrome		17
FGFR2	10q26	Crouzon, Pfeiffer & Apert syndromes		17
FGFR3	4p16.3	Coronal craniosynostosis		17,18
TWIST	7p21	Saethre-Chotzen syndrome		17,19

The critical events in craniofacial patterning, from the trilaminar
embryo to a miniature identifiable human, take place within a
remarkably short time window, from 19 to 50 days post-conception
(one calendar month). It is important to note that gastrulation
and neurulation occur during the first week after the missed men-
strual period. This emphasises both the need for pre-conception
folic acid supplementation to reduce the risk of neural tube defect
and the danger of teratogens (notably alcohol) in the newly
pregnant but potentially unaware mother.

Holoprosencephaly and sonic hedgehog: when genetics really works...

Holoprosencephaly (HPE) comprises a spectrum of malformations
resulting from deficiency of midline facial structures, with an

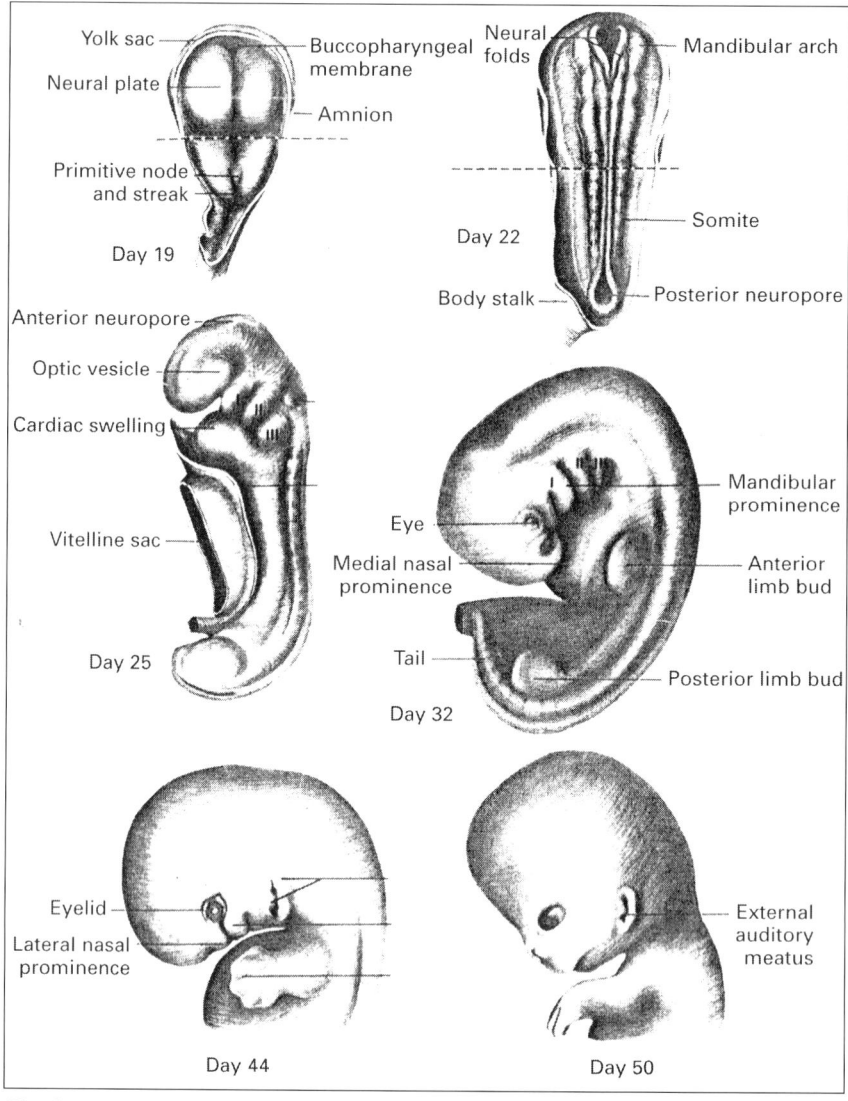

Fig 2. *Development of the human embryo from the germ layer stage (day 19) to near the end of the embryonic period (day 50).* Particular features to note are the neural plate (day 19), formation of neural tube with migration of neural crest cells (days 22 and 25), and development of facial swellings (days 32 and 44). Mineralisation of the skull vault does not start until about 13 weeks (ca day 50). (Reprinted with permission from Ref 24.)

estimated prevalence of one in 250 induced abortions and one in 16,000 live births. An important non-genetic cause in both human and mouse is alcohol ingestion. Extrapolation from studies in mice suggests that HPE arises in the third week of pregnancy from deficiency of the midline part of the anterior neural plate (reviewed in Ref 25).

Clinically, the HPE spectrum is very variable. In the mildest form, the only sign may be the presence of a single midline central incisor. The most severe forms, universally lethal, are characterised by cyclopia (a single, central eye), absence of the nose, central proboscis and fusion of the forebrain.

As described elsewhere in this book, four general approaches may be used to identify disease genes:

- chromosomal abnormalities,
- genetic linkage analysis,
- candidate genes, and
- animal models.

HPE provides a beautiful example of a disorder in which all four approaches contributed to the identification of mutations in a gene called sonic hedgehog (*SHH*). The first clue to gene localisation came in the 1980s when microdeletions and translocations in sporadic cases of HPE were identified in several chromosomal regions, including 2p, 7q, 18p and 21q. Subsequently, linkage analysis in families segregating autosomal dominant HPE gave significant positive logarithm of the odds (LOD) scores to polymorphic markers on 7q36, confirming this localisation.

Sonic hedgehog gene

SHH was originally identified in vertebrates by cross-hybridisation at reduced stringency to the *hedgehog* gene from *Drosophila* (the 'sonic' epithet differentiates it from two other vertebrate *hedgehog* paralogues, and reflects the discoverers' warped sense of humour). Initially, two lines of evidence suggested that *SHH* could be an HPE gene:

- it was shown to be expressed in the midline (node and noto-chord) in early embryogenesis,[2] and
- it mapped to chromosome band 7q36.

The suspicion was strengthened when a mouse 'knock-out' for the *shh* gene was constructed: the homozygous null embryos died around birth with cyclopia and a proboscis.[3] Subsequently, two reports confirmed that heterozygous mutations of *SHH* were present in some patients with HPE.[4,5] The *SHH* mutations occur on only one allele and are predicted to cause loss of function, so the disease mechanism is described as haploinsufficiency. For most proteins, a 50% reduction would not matter, but it seems that critical developmental regulators are quite commonly dosage sensitive.[26]

Function of the SHH protein

What does the SHH protein actually do? In *Drosophila*, it is known to be a secreted molecule involved in cell-cell communication, signalling to cellular targets by a complex mechanism requiring binding to a transmembrane protein called patched (PTCH). Intriguingly, a mammalian orthologue of PTCH has also been identified, heterozygous mutations of which have been identified in an entirely different syndrome, the basal cell naevus or Gorlin syndrome.[6] Yet another participant in the hedgehog signalling pathway, GLI3 (Table 1), is mutated in Greig cephalopolysyndactyly[7,8] and other phenotypes.

Although this example has been chosen as a compelling vindication of the genetic approach to craniofacial malformation, several pieces of the HPE/SHH story in the landmark publications[4,5] actually did not fit neatly into place. These exceptions emphasise that finding disease genes is the beginning, not the end, in the goal of understanding pathogenesis:

- In contrast to the human, heterozygotes for the mouse *shh* 'knock-out' are phenotypically normal. It is perhaps not surprising that the mouse is not always a perfect model of the human condition.[27]
- None of four chromosomal translocations of 7q36 associated with HPE disrupt the *SHH* gene,[4] which at one stage led researchers to discount a role for SHH. It is presumed that these translocations affect *SHH* expression through a 'position effect'.[28]
- Occasional individuals carrying mutations of *SHH* are phenotypically normal – an example of non-penetrance.[5] Differences in phenotype between family members inheriting the same mutation are generally attributed to differences in genetic and environmental background.

Branchial arch disorders: novel genes and stochastic events

As shown in Fig 2, the branchial arches, the embryological equivalent of the gills in fish, form during the fourth week partly by the migration of neural crest cells. They contribute to various structures in the head and neck, including the facial skeleton, hyoid bone and larynx.

Treacher Collins syndrome

Treacher Collins syndrome (prevalence one in 50,000) is an auto-somal dominant disorder comprising symmetrical mandibular and zygomatic hypoplasia, lower eyelid coloboma, rudimentary ears, deafness and cleft palate. A similar phenotype can be induced by exposure of mouse embryos to retinoic acid, leading to the sug-gestion that the regional deficiencies are secondary to excessive cell death around the trigeminal ganglionic placode (reviewed in Refs 12 and 25).

Genetic linkage of Treacher Collins syndrome to 5q was originally established in 1991[29] but, in contrast to HPE and 7q, none of the obvious candidate genes in the region turned out to be correct. The responsible gene, termed *TCOF1*, was eventually identified in 1996 following a heroic effort in positional cloning.[11] No gene equivalent to *TCOF1* had previously been identified in any species, although its sequence shows similarity to nucleolar phosphoproteins. Preliminary expression studies in the mouse show high levels in the first and second branchial arches, as well as in many other embryonic and adult tissues.[12] In this case, human genetics has revealed an entirely new molecule for the developmental biologists to study.

Hemifacial microsomia

The abnormalities in hemifacial microsomia, part of the oculo-auriculo-vertebral spectrum (prevalence one in 5,600), may superficially resemble those of Treacher Collins syndrome but are often asymmetrical and occurrence is usually sporadic (recurrence risk for siblings: 2–3%). Mandibular hypoplasia is frequently associ-ated with absence of the temporo-mandibular joint, microtia and ear tags. Poswillo[30] originally showed that a similar spectrum of abnormalities could be obtained in mice and macaques by inducing haemorrhage in the embryonic stapedial artery.

More recently, a mouse mutant, *Hfm*, has been described.[31] This arose by the random insertion of a transgene construct into mouse chromosome 10. About 25% of mice inheriting the transgene develop microtia and other asymmetric facial abnormalities, and the other 75% are normal. Examination of day 10 mouse embryos reveals rupture of vessels in the second branchial arch, usually unilaterally, in a minority. It seems that the transgene integration selectively predisposes to these haemorrhages by an unknown mechanism. The expanding haematoma disorganises the mesenchyme in a localised area of the face, without respecting embryological boundaries. Presumably, the phenotype is penetrant only if this event occurs during a critical developmental window (equivalent to the fifth week in man), dependent on stochastic (ie chance) factors, and perhaps on genetic and environmental background. Although the *Hfm* locus has not yet been identified, the presence of the transgene should provide an excellent molecular 'handle' to home in on the responsible gene.

Craniosynostosis: a conserved developmental pathway from flies to man?

Craniosynostosis (prevalence one in 2,100) describes the premature fusion of the cranial sutures, the sites where growth of the skull normally occurs. It is a much later event than any of those described above. Ossification of the skull, which occurs directly in mesenchynal connective tissue rather than through a cartilage intermediate, does not start until 13 weeks of gestation and the bone fronts meet to form sutures at about 18 weeks. A large number of craniosynostosis syndromes have been described, many of which are differentiated by the pattern of involvement of the limbs. This clinical genetic observation suggests a close tie-up between some processes of cranial and limb development.

Fibroblast growth factor receptor mutations

Missense mutations of fibroblast growth factor (FGF) receptors, FGFR1, 2 and 3 have been identified in six autosomal dominant craniosynostosis syndromes since 1994.[17] The best known of these are the Pfeiffer (Fig 1), Crouzon and Apert syndromes. More recently, a single, specific mutation of *FGFR3* was shown to account for about 30% of patients with apparently non-syndromic craniosynostosis.[18] Different mutations of *FGFR3* have been described in several chondrodysplasia syndromes, including achondroplasia.[32] FGFRs are cell membrane proteins that signal the presence of extracellular FGFs to the inside of the cell. In contrast to the loss-of-function effects of SHH and TCOF1 mutations, specific FGFR mutations appear to activate the receptor[17,32] by a variety of different gain-of-function mechanisms, which is one reason why different mutations of the same protein can result in diverse phenotypes.

Mutations of TWIST, a transcription factor

In 1997, mutations of a very different gene, the transcription factor *TWIST*, were identified in another cause of craniosynostosis, Saethre-Chotzen syndrome. *TWIST* is another gene originally isolated in *Drosophila*, in which it serves as a master regulator activating a cascade of genetic pathways in mesoderm formation. One of its targets is an FGFR; perhaps the equivalent pathway is conserved in vertebrate cranial suture differentiation.[17,19]

Cleft lip/palate

Varied aetiology, complex genetics

Clefts of the lip and/or palate have two distinct embryological origins:

- *Primary palate defects* (prevalence one in 500 to one in 1,000) result from incomplete fusion of the intermaxillary and maxillary processes at about 6–7 weeks and cause cleft lip with or without cleft palate (CL±P).
- *Cleft palate* alone (CP) (prevalence one in 2,500) is pathologically distinct, arises later in development (7–10 weeks), and is caused by failure of the palatal shelves to elevate and fuse.

Both defects occur secondary to maxillary tissue deficiency or dysmorphogenesis arising from a wide diversity of genetic or environmental insults.

Syndromic clefts comprise about 30% of the total. Identified genetic causes of CL±P include chromosomal abnormalities such as trisomy 13 and monosomy 4p as well as the single gene disorder Opitz G syndrome (Table 1). Stickler syndrome (Table 1) and 22q11 deletion (DiGeorge velocardiofacial syndrome[33] are important causes of CP. Many cases have complex aetiology and various attempts have been made to map polygenes involved in CL±P. Although linkage and association studies have identified various promising candidate genes (including *BCL1*, *END1*, *RARA* and *TGFA*), it has been difficult to obtain consistently positive results with any of these.[34]

Fetal protein therapy for craniofacial disorders

Even the most enthusiastic proponents of gene therapy would agree that craniofacial disorders do not seem attractive targets for intervention. Many are dominantly inherited, implying that presence of one normal gene copy does not prevent the malformation occurring, and all would require treatment in fetal life. It therefore comes as a surprise that a 'cure' by fetal protein therapy has been claimed for one mouse model of cleft palate. The transforming growth factor (*TGF*) β3 gene is expressed precisely along the midline seam of the fusing palatal shelves, and two groups have shown that homozygous deficiency of *TGFβ3* in mice results in CP.[35,36] This defect can be corrected *in vitro* by treatment of palatal cultures with TGFβ3 protein,[37] and recent unpublished data from Ferguson's group indicate that *in vivo* correction (by injection of the pregnant mother) is also successful. Until a pathophysiological role for TGFβ3 in human CP can be clearly established, however, it is doubtful whether this technical *tour de force* could be applied clinically.

Conclusion

As shown in Table 2, the genes mutated in craniofacial disorders encode a wide variety of proteins, including signalling molecules, receptors, transcription factors and structural proteins. The mutations may cause either gain-of-function (structural disruption or

Table 2. Genes and molecular pathogenesis in craniofacial disorders.
Cellular function may be perturbed at any stage from cell-cell signalling, through signal transduction and activation of transcription factors, to synthesis of structural proteins (classification of molecular mechanism from Ref 26).

Gene	Function	Molecular mechanism
SHH	Secreted protein	Haploinsufficiency
FGFR1		
FGFR2	Signal transduction	Constitutive activation
FGFR3		
MSX2		Increased DNA binding
GLI3		
PAX3	Transcription factor	
OSF2/CBFA1		Haploinsufficiency
TWIST		
MID1		
EYA1	Transcription factor?	
COL2A1		
COL11A1	Structural protein	Disrupted structure
COL11A2		
TCOF1	Nucleolar phosphoprotein	Dominant negative?

constitutive activation) or loss-of-function (haploinsufficiency or position effect). Identification of disease causing mutations enables much more precise genetic counselling for affected families and provides entirely new leads towards understanding the pathogenesis.

Progress in identifying further disease genes is likely to be rapid. Spurred by these developments, at least one research group is even initiating attempts to identify genes involved in normal facial characteristics. It remains an open question whether the disease genes described in this chapter will turn out to contribute.

Acknowledgements

I am grateful to David Johnson for reading the manuscript, and to Sir David Weatherall for support. Work in my laboratory is funded by the Wellcome Trust.

References

1 Marden PM, Smith DW, McDonald MJ. Congenital anomalies in the newborn infant, including minor variations. *Journal of Pediatrics* 1964; **64**: 357–71.

2 Echelard Y, Epstein DJ, St-Jacques B, Shen L, *et al.* Sonic hedgehog, a member of a family of putative signaling molecules, is implicated in the regulation of CNS polarity. *Cell* 1993; **75**: 1417–30.

3 Chiang C, Litingtung Y, Lee E, Young KE, *et al.* Cyclopia and defective axial patterning in mice lacking *sonic hedgehog* gene function. *Nature* 1996; **383**: 407–13.

4 Belloni E, Muenke M, Roessler E, Traverso G, *et al.* Identification of *sonic hedgehog* as a candidate gene responsible for holoprosencephaly. *Nature Genetics* 1996; **14**: 353–6.

5 Roessler E, Belloni E, Gaudenz K, Jay P, *et al.* Mutations in the human *sonic hedgehog* gene cause holoprosencephaly. *Nature Genetics* 1996; **14**: 357–60.

6 McMahon AP, Chuan P-T. Hedgehogs in the clinic. *Nature Medicine* 1996; **2**: 1308–10.

7 Hui C-C, Joyner AL. A mouse model of Greig cephalopolysyndactyly syndrome: the *extra-toes* mutation contains an intragenic deletion of the *Gli3* gene. *Nature Genetics* 1993; **3**: 241–6.

8 Wild A, Kalff-Suske M, Vortkamp A, Bornholdt D, *et al.* Point mutations in human *GLI3* cause Greig syndrome. *Human Molecular Genetics* 1997; **6**: 1979–84.

9 Quaderi NA, Schweiger S, Gaudenz K, Franco B, *et al.* Opitz G/BBB syndrome, a defect of midline development, is due to mutations in a new RING finger gene on Xp22. *Nature Genetics* 1997; **17**: 285–91.

10 Read AP, Newton VE. Waardenburg syndrome. *Journal of Medical Genetics* 1997; **34**: 656–65.

11   The Treacher Collins Syndrome Collaborative Group. Positional
     cloning of a gene involved in the pathogenesis of Treacher Collins
     syndrome. *Nature Genetics* 1996; **12**: 130–6.
12   Dixon J, Hovanes K, Shiang R, Dixon MJ. Sequence analysis, identifi-
     cation of evolutionary conserved motifs and expression analysis of
     murine tcof1 provide further evidence for a potential function for
     the gene and its human homologue TCOF1. *Human Molecular
     Genetics* 1997; **6**: 727–37.
13   Abdelhak S, Kalatzis V, Heilig R, Compain S, *et al.* A human
     homologue of the *Drosophila eyes absent* gene underlines branchio-
     oto-renal (BOR) syndrome and identifies a novel gene family. *Nature
     Genetics* 1997; **15**: 157–64.
14   Vikkula M, Mariman ECM, Lui VCH, Zhidkova NI, *et al.* Autosomal
     dominant and recessive osteochondrodysplasias associated with the
     COL11A2 locus. *Cell* 1995; **80**: 431–7.
15   Richards AJ, Yates JRW, Williams R, Payne SJ, *et al.* A family with
     Stickler syndrome type 2 has a mutation in the *COL11A1* gene result-
     ing in the substitution of glycine 97 by valine in α(XI) collagen.
     Human Molecular Genetics 1996; **5**: 1339–43.
16   Rodan GA, Harada S-I. The missing bone. *Cell* 1997; **89**: 677–80.
17   Wilkie AOM. Craniosynostosis: genes and mechanisms. *Human
     Molecular Genetics* 1997; **6**: 1647–56.
18   Moloney DM, Wall SA, Ashworth GJ, Oldridge M, *et al.* Prevalence of
     Pro250Arg mutation of fibroblast growth factor receptor 3 in coronal
     craniosynostosis. *Lancet* 1997; **349**: 1059–62.
19   Rose CSP, Malcolm S. A TWIST in development. *Trends in Genetics*
     1997; **13**: 384–7.
20   Winter RM. What's in a face? *Nature Genetics* 1996; **12**: 124–9.
21   Gorlin RJ, Cohen MM Jr, Levin LS. *Syndromes of the head and neck.* New
     York: Oxford University Press, 1990.
22   Noden DM. Interactions and fates of avian craniofacial mesenchyme.
     Development 1988; **103**: 121–40.
23   Couly GF, Coltey PM, Le Douarin NM. The triple origin of skull in
     higher vertebrates: a study in quail-chick chimeras. *Development* 1993;
     117: 409–29.
24   Johnston MC, Sulik KK. Development of the face and oral cavity. In:
     Bhaskar SN (ed). *Orban's oral histology and embryology,* 11th edn. St
     Louis, MO: CV Mosby, 1991: 2.
25   Johnston MC. Understanding human embryonic development. In:
     Stevenson RE, Hall JG, Goodman RM (eds). *Human malformations
     and related anomalies.* New York: Oxford University Press, 1993: 31–63.
26   Wilkie AOM. The molecular basis of genetic dominance. *Journal of
     Medical Genetics* 1994; **31**: 89–98.
27   Wynshaw-Boris A. Model mice and human disease. *Nature Genetics*
     1996; **13**: 259–60.
28   Bedell MA, Jenkins NA, Copeland NG. Good genes in bad neighbour-
     hoods. *Nature Genetics* 1996; **12**: 229–32.
29   Dixon MJ, Read AP, Donnai D, Colley A, *et al.* The gene for Treacher
     Collins syndrome maps to the long arm of chromosome 5. *American
     Journal of Human Genetics* 1991; **49**: 17–22.

30 Poswillo D. The aetiology and pathogenesis of craniofacial deformity. *Development* 1988; **103** (Suppl): 207–12.

31 Naora H, Kimura M, Otani H, Yokoyama M, *et al.* Transgenic mouse model of hemifacial microsomia: cloning and characterization of insertional mutation region on chromosome 10. *Genomics* 1994; **23**: 515–9.

32 Webster MK, Donoghue DJ. FGFR activation in skeletal disorders: too much of a good thing. *Trends in Genetics* 1997; **13**: 178–82.

33 Ryan AK, Goodship JA, Wilson DI, Philip N, *et al.* Spectrum of clinical features associated with interstitial chromosome 22q11 deletions: a European collaborative study. *Journal of Medical Genetics* 1997; **34**: 798–804.

34 Murray JC. Face facts: genes, environments, and clefts. *American Journal of Human Genetics* 1995; **57**: 227–32.

35 Proetzel G, Pawlowski SA, Wiles MV, Yin M, *et al.* Transforming growth factor-β3 is required for secondary palate fusion. *Nature Genetics* 1995; **11**: 409–14.

36 Kaartinen V, Voncken JW, Shuler C, Warburton D, *et al.* Abnormal lung development and cleft palate in mice lacking TGF-β3 indicates defects of epithelial-mesenchymal interaction. *Nature Genetics* 1995; **11**: 415–21.

37 Taya Y, O'Kane S, Ferguson MWJ. Rescue of cleft palate in TGF-β3 knockout mice in vitro. *Developmental Biology* 1997; **186**: 270.

9 | Tuberous sclerosis

Andrew J Green
National Centre for Medical Genetics,
University College Dublin,
Our Lady's Hospital for Sick Children, Dublin

Clinical manifestations

Tuberous sclerosis (TSC) is an autosomal dominant condition characterised by benign tumour-like malformations (hamartomas) of the skin, brain, heart, kidney and other organs. The disease prevalence is estimated at a minimum of one in 10,000, two-thirds of the cases being sporadic and representing new dominant mutation.[1] It was first described by von Recklinghausen in the 19th century, and has had the eponyms of Bournville or Pringle disease. In the past, Vogt's triad of mental retardation, seizures and 'adenoma sebaceum' defined the clinical diagnosis, but it is now becoming clear that TSC has a far wider range of manifestations, with many cases of TSC not fitting into the classical disease. With the recognition of the highly varied expression of TSC, Gomez and Roach have coined the term 'tuberous sclerosis complex'.[1,2]

Brain manifestations

About half the patients with TSC have significant mental handicap, and those with handicap almost always have seizures. The classic presentation of seizures in TSC is infantile spasms, which are a poor prognostic feature. However, some people with TSC may have only a few seizures and no intellectual impairment. Abnormal behaviour patterns, often with autistic tendencies, are frequently a manifestation of the condition.

On pathological examination, the brain contains multiple tubers, dysplastic areas of tissue with loss of the delineation between grey and white matter. The number of tubers does not necessarily correlate with the severity of brain involvement, but there is evidence to suggest that the site of the tubers may determine behavioural abnormalities. There may be small nodules of tissue on the subependymal surface of the ventricles of the brain, which can often calcify. Benign tumours may also occur in the intraventricular spaces (these have been called giant cell astrocytomas) and can cause hydrocephalus if they block the flow of cerebrospinal fluid.

Skin signs

Almost all those with TSC have signs on their skin, but such signs can be quite subtle. The hypopigmented patches may often be missed, and the skin should be examined under ultraviolet light to detect the 'ash-leaf patch' – which, in reality, frequently bears no resemblance to any leaf. The old term, 'adenoma sebaceum', used to describe the facial lesions, is incorrect as the lesions are in fact angiofibromas and do not arise from sebaceous glands. A shagreen patch in the lumbar region is typical in TSC, as are multiple nail fibromas.

Cardiac and renal symptoms

About half of all infants with TSC will have multiple cardiac rhabdomyomas at birth; these rarely cause symptoms and disappear in the first few years of life. About half of all patients with TSC will develop multiple renal angiomyolipomas, usually from their teenage years onwards, but only a small number of them will become symptomatic with loin pain or haemorrhage from the lesions. Renal cysts can also occur, and renal cell carcinoma is rare but recognised.

Other organ involvement

Other organs can be involved, such as the retina, gums or colon. A retinal phakoma is histologically identical to the giant cell astrocytoma seen in the brain, and rarely causes visual disturbance. It can be mistaken on fundoscopy for a retinoblastoma, but has an innocent course and only occasionally needs removal. Gum fibromas and dental pits are found in the mouth, colonic polyps have also been seen, and hepatic angiomyolipomas occur but are not usually problematic.

Clinical genetics

About 60–70% of those with TSC are born to unaffected parents and represent new autosomal dominant mutations, but there are also autosomal dominant families and the disease can show a wide range of expression within the same family. When a child is found to have TSC, both parents should be examined carefully for any clinical signs of the condition. It is not uncommon to find clear signs of TSC in a parent who had never previously considered himself or herself to be affected. A computed tomography scan of the brain and a renal ultrasound may help to clarify an asymptomatic parent's status. It is also not uncommon to find families in which one parent may show some clinical sign suggestive of TSC, which in itself would not be of significance but raises concerns when that person has a child affected with TSC.

Where neither parent of a child with TSC shows any signs of the condition, there is about a 3% chance of another child being affected with TSC. Families with two affected children born to normal parents are recognised, and may represent mosaicism for a TSC gene mutation in one of the parents. Where a parent is affected with TSC, each child has a 50% chance of also being affected, but it is currently not possible to predict the degree to which that child might be affected.

Molecular genetics

The search for the tuberous sclerosis genes

The first description of linkage in TSC was in 1987 for markers on chromosome 9q34, and a long hunt for the *TSC1* gene began.[3] It later became apparent that some families did not show linkage to 9q34. Loci on chromosomes 11 and 12 were suggested, but have now been discounted. In 1992, a second locus for *TSC, TSC2*, was described on chromosome 16p13.3, using the same markers as had been used for the polycystic kidney disease (PKD) gene, *PKD1*.[4] This raised the possibility that PKD and TSC might be allelic, as the former is well recognised in TSC. The TSC1 and TSC2 loci each account for about 50% of familial TSC cases, and there are no clear clinical differences between families linked to either locus (see Fig 1).[5]

The presence of multiple hamartomas in several organs in TSC suggested that the *TSC* genes might each act as a form of tumour suppressor, similar to the model proposed by Knudson.[6] In this model, an inactivating mutation is present in the germline copy of a tumour suppressor gene (*TSG*). An inactivating mutation of the second normal allele of that gene in any cell will then be sufficient

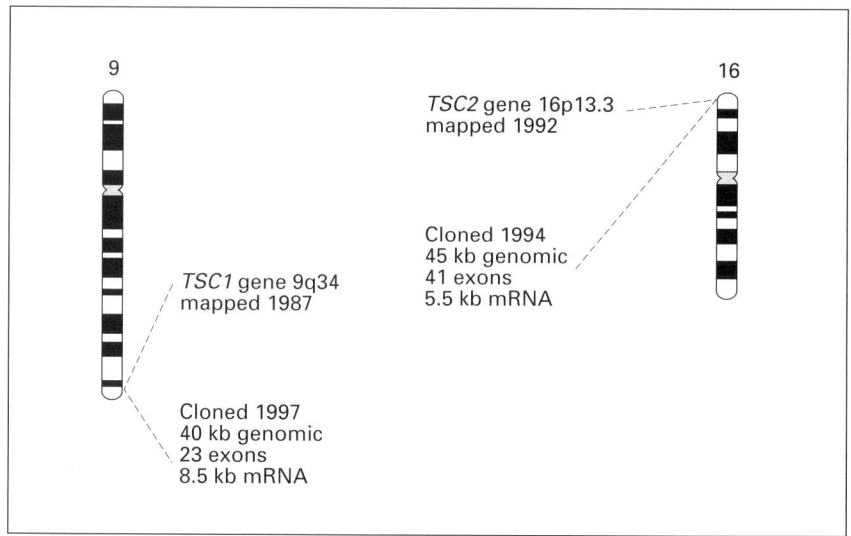

Fig 1. *Tuberous sclerosis complex (TSC) genes.*

to allow its proliferation as a tumour. This model describes the mutation as dominant in the germline, but recessive at the cellular level. The hallmark of a *TSG* is the loss of heterozygosity (LOH) of a polymorphic DNA marker in the region of the putative *TSG*. LOH is likely to represent one mechanism of inactivating a somatic allele of a *TSG*. Such LOH has been found in six different types of TSC hamartoma, and is more frequent in the region of the *TSC2* than the *TSC1* gene.[7-11]

Characterisation of the TSC2 gene

The *TSC2* gene was characterised in 1993, and intragenic deletions of 1–5 kb have been identified in this gene in a small number of cases of TSC.[12] These deletions can involve the adjacent *PKD1* gene, and are then associated with significant cystic renal disease.[13] The *TSC2* gene product has been named tuberin, and is encoded by a ubiquitously expressed 5.5 kb mRNA. The gene spans approximately 45 kb of genomic DNA and is made up of 41 exons. These exons vary in size from 70–213 bp, with one larger exon of 488 bp.[14] A region of 58 amino acids towards the C-terminal of the predicted TSC2 protein shows similarity to the GTPase-activating protein (GAP) 3.[12] The expressed TSC2 protein interacts with an intracellular GTPase, rab5.[15] Small intragenic TSC2 mutations have also been found, the majority of which are predicted to cause a non-functional protein. All the mutations appear to be specific to each family, but even in families with linkage to *TSC2* not all the expected mutations have been detected.[16-20] Missense mutations in the GAP3-related domain also appear to be pathogenic.[21] The detection rate for TSC2 mutations, using reverse transcriptase polymerase chain reaction of TSC2 mRNA from lymphocytes (with either protein truncation assays or single-strand conformation analysis) is 28–30%.[20,22] Both somatic and germ-cell mosaicism for TSC2 gene mutations has been described,[17,23] and the molecular confirmation of TSC2 gene mosaicism will make counselling more rather than less difficult in the future.

The Eker rat, a dominantly inherited renal cancer syndrome, is a naturally occurring TSC2 gene mutant. An insertional mutation into the rat *TSC2* gene causes the condition, second somatic TSC2 mutations in renal cell cancers occur, and transfection of the wild type rat *TSC2* gene rescues the phenotype of the cancer cells.[24-26] This condition does not, however, closely resemble human TSC, although renal cell cancer can occur in humans with TSC.

Isolation of the TSC1 gene

As the result of a concerted effort by a consortium of six research groups, the *TSC1* gene has recently been isolated by a combination of positional cloning and large-scale sequencing.[27] The gene lies between the anonymous markers D9S1830 and D9S1199, and spans an area of 40 kb. It has an 8.5 kb mRNA encoded by 23 exons, 21 of which code for the TSC1 protein, hamartin, which has a predicted mass of 130 kD and contains 1,164 amino acids. The TSC1 gene product has no homology to known proteins, including the *TSC2* gene, but does contain a coiled-coil domain.

In contrast to the *TSC2* gene, no large germline deletions were found in TSC patients. Eight of the 21 coding exons were analysed, and 42 mutations found in a large panel of cases of TSC. Almost all the mutations were predicted to give rise to a truncated protein, with the mutation 2105delAAAG a recurrent mutation seen in six independent cases. The other mutations appear to be private to each family. The largest exon, exon 15 (500 bp), contained 23 mutations, and 19 mutations were found in the other seven exons analysed. One sporadic case with a germline 2105delAAAG mutation had a second somatic truncating mutation in a renal cell carcinoma, strongly suggesting that the *TSC1* gene also acts as a tumour suppressor.

Two other cases with germline mutations had previously been shown to have LOH in hamartomas for the *TSC1* region,[11] in one of which the germline mutant allele was retained. Analysis by single-strand conformation polymorphism of the complete genomic coding region of the *TSC1* gene in a group of 81 patients gave a detection rate of 19% for mutations (unpublished personal data). Almost all these mutations are predicted to give a truncated TSC1 protein.

Future developments

The cloning of the *TSC1* gene and the improvement in mutation detection technology may now make molecular diagnosis in TSC more feasible. Such molecular detection is likely to clarify the situation for those families where the uncertainty of the origin of a TSC gene mutation is a pressing clinical issue. Several projects are now under way to assess the clinical usefulness of *TSC* gene mutation detection.

As with the cloning of any disease gene, the finding of the *TSC1* and *TSC2* genes opens up many opportunities for the study of the cell biology of both genes. The *TSC2* gene appears to play a role in intracellular compartments through its interaction with rab5. Knock-out studies of both genes in transgenic animals may provide a model of the human disease and the opportunity to study the interaction between both genes *in vivo*. Further understanding of the biology of the *TSC2* gene will also give insights into the pathogenesis of hamartomas. Similar developments are eagerly awaited for the TSC1 gene product.

References

1 Gomez MR. Phenotypes of the tuberous sclerosis complex with a revision of diagnostic criteria. *Annals of the New York Academy of Sciences* 1991; **615**: 1–7.
2 Roach ES. International tuberous sclerosis conference (editorial). *Journal of Child Neurology* 1990; **5**: 269–72.
3 Fryer AE, Connor JM, Povey S, Yates JRW, *et al*. Evidence that the gene for tuberous sclerosis is on chromosome 9. *Lancet* 1987; **i**: 659–61.
4 Kandt RS, Haines JL, Smith M, Northrup H, *et al*. Linkage of an important gene locus for tuberous sclerosis to a chromosome 16 marker for polycystic kidney disease. *Nature Genetics* 1992; **2**: 37–41.
5 Burley MW, Attwood J, Benham F, Fairbrother U, *et al*. *Linkage studies in tuberous sclerosis*. Second International Chromosome 9 Workshop, Chatham, NY, USA, 1993: 10.
6 Knudson AGJ. Mutation and cancer: statistical study of retinoblastoma. *Proceedings of the National Academy of Sciences of the USA* 1971; **68**: 820–3.

7 Green AJ, Smith M, Yates JRW. Loss of heterozygosity on chromosome 16p13.3 in hamartomas from tuberous sclerosis patients. *Nature Genetics* 1994; **6**: 193–6.

8 Green AJ, Johnson PH, Yates JRW. The tuberous sclerosis gene on chromosome 9q34 acts as a growth suppressor. *Human Molecular Genetics* 1994; **3**: 1833–4.

9 Carbonara C, Longa L, Grosso E, Borone C, *et al.* 9q34 loss of heterozygosity in a tuberous sclerosis astrocytoma suggests a growth suppressor-like activity also for the TSCl gene. *Human Molecular Genetics* 1994; **3**: 1829–32.

10 Carbonara C, Longa L, Grosso E, Mazzacco G, *et al.* Apparent preferential loss of heterozygosity at *TSC2* over *TSC1* chromosomal region in tuberous sclerosis hamartomas. *Genes, Chromosomes and Cancer* 1996; **15**: 18–25.

11 Sepp T, Yates JR, Green AJ. Loss of heterozygosity in tuberous sclerosis hamartomas. *Journal of Medical Genetics* 1996; **33**: 962.

12 The European Chromosome 16 Tuberous Sclerosis Consortium. Identification and characterisation of the tuberous sclerosis gene on chromosome 16. *Cell* 1993; **75**: 1–11.

13 Brook-Carter PT, Peral B, Ward CJ, Thompson P, *et al.* Deletion of the *TSC2* and PKD1 genes associated with severe infantile polycystic kidney disease – a contiguous gene syndrome. *Nature Genetics* 1994; **8**: 328–32.

14 Maheshwar MM, Sandford R, Nellist M, Cheadle JP, *et al.* Comparative analysis and genomic structure of the tuberous sclerosis 2 (*TSC2*) gene in human and pufferfish. *Human Molecular Genetics* 1996; **5**: 131–7.

15 Xiao G-H, Shoarinejad F, Jin F, Golemis EA, Yeung RS. The tuberous sclerosis 2 gene product, tuberin, functions as a Rab5 GTPase activating protein (GAP) in modulating endocytosis. *Journal of Biological Chemistry* 1997; **272**: 6097–100.

16 Vrtel R, Verhoef S, Bouman K, Maheshwar MM, *et al.* Identification of a nonsense mutation at the 5'-end of the *TSC2* gene in a family with a presumptive diagnosis of tuberous sclerosis complex. *Journal of Medical Genetics* 1996; **33**: 47–51.

17 Verhoef S, Vrtel R, van Essen T, Bakker L, *et al.* Somatic mosaicism and clinical variation in tuberous sclerosis complex (letter). *Lancet* 1995; **345**: 202.

18 Kumar A, Kandt RS, Wolpert C, Roses AD, *et al.* Mutation analysis of the *TSC2* gene in an African-American family. *Human Molecular Genetics* 1995; **4**: 2295–8.

19 Kumar A, Wolpert C, Kandt RS, Segal J, *et al.* A de novo frame-shift mutation in the tuberin gene. *Human Molecular Genetics* 1995; **4**: 1471–2.

20 Wilson PJ, Ramesh V, Kristiansen A, Boue C, *et al.* Novel mutations detected in the TSC2 gene from both sporadic and familial TSC patients. *Human Molecular Genetics* 1996; **5**: 249–56.

21 Maheshwar M, Chealde J, Jones A, Myring J, *et al.* The GAP-related domain of tuberin, the product of the *TSC2* gene, is a target for missense mutations in tuberous sclerosis. *Human Molecular Genetics* 1997; **6**: 1991–6.

22 van Bakel I, Sepp T, Ward S, Yates JR, Green AJ. Mutations in the *TSC2* gene: analysis of the complete coding sequence using the protein truncation test (PTT). *Human Molecular Genetics* 1997; **6**: 1409–14.

23 Yates J, van Bakel I, Sepp T, Payne S. Female germline mosaicism in tuberous sclerosis. *Human Molecular Genetics* 1997; **6**: 2265–9.

24 Yeung RS, Xiao GH, Jin F, Lee WC, *et al.* Predisposition to renal carcinoma in the Eker rat is determined by germ-line mutation of the tuberous sclerosis 2 (*TSC2*) gene. *Proceedings of the National Academy of Sciences of the USA* 1994; **91**: 11413–6.

25 Yeung RS, Xiao GH, Everitt JI, Jin F, Walker CL. Allelic loss at the tuberous sclerosis 2 locus in spontaneous tumors in the Eker rat. *Molecular Carcinogenesis* 1995; **14**: 28–36.

26 Orimoto K, Tsuchiya H, Kobayashi T, Matsuda T, Hino O. Suppression of the neoplastic phenotype by replacement of the *TSC2* gene in Eker rat renal carcinoma cells. *Biochemical and Biophysical Research Communications* 1996; **219**: 70–5.

27 van Slegtenhorst M, de Hoogt R, Hermans C, Nellist M, *et al.* Identification of the tuberous sclerosis gene *TSC1* on chromosome 9q34. *Science* 1997; **277**: 805–8.

10 | A molecular update on autosomal dominant polycystic kidney disease

Peter C Harris

MRC Molecular Haematology Unit, Institute of Molecular Medicine, University of Oxford

The autosomal dominant form of polycystic kidney disease (ADPKD) is one of the commonest single gene disorders. It has an estimated frequency of one in 1,000 individuals affected, and there are reported cases in most human populations. It is of considerable clinical importance, being responsible for about 8% of patients with end-stage renal disease (ESRD) (those requiring dialysis or transplantation). The name by which it is often known, adult polycystic kidney disease, indicates that this is usually a late onset disorder. Polycystic kidney disease (PKD) manifesting in childhood has traditionally been considered to be due to the rarer autosomal recessive form of PKD, which is often called infantile PKD. However, in recent years it has become clear that there is considerable phenotypic variability in the severity of renal disease in ADPKD. Although about 25% of patients still have adequate renal function at 70 years,[1] analysis of childhood PKD shows that more than a quarter are early manifestation of the dominant form of the disease.[2]

Clinical spectrum

The major cause of morbidity and mortality in ADPKD is the progressive formation and growth of multiple fluid-filled cysts leading to bilateral PKD. During this process, the normal precise architecture of the kidney (ca 1 million nephrons) is replaced with an enlarged structure consisting of thousands of cysts varying in size from less than 1 mm to more than 10 cm. Cysts are also found in many other organs, with massive cystic disease of the liver a rare complication of clinical significance, most often found in females.[3]

The systemic nature of ADPKD is further illustrated by associations with a variety of non-cystic lesions. Of greatest clinical significance is an increased prevalence of intracranial berry aneurysms that can rupture, resulting in subarachnoid haemorrhage. The prevalence of this complication has been estimated as 1–37%, with evidence of familial clustering.[1] An association has also been noted with a variety of other disorders of connective tissue including heart valve defects, inguinal hernia and colonic diverticula,[5] with rarely a Marfanoid habitus described.[6] These clinical manifestations indicate that the ADPKD protein(s) play a role beyond the kidney.

Cyst formation

Careful microdissection of ADPKD kidneys at an early stage of the disease has shown that only a small proportion of nephrons (ca 1%) become cystic, and that cysts develop as focal dilations or outpouchings of the tubule.[7,8] Although cysts are thought to form from all regions of the nephron in ADPKD, staining suggests that in adult disease the majority arise from distal tubules and the collecting duct. These focal tubular dilations are not associated with tubule blockage, but at an early stage the epithelia appear to be simplified and dedifferentiated, and the associated basement membrane (BM) thickened and disorganised. Noting these changes early in cystogenesis, the primary defect(s) in this disorder have variously been suggested as:

- a factor controlling epithelial cell differentiation,
- a component of the BM, or
- disruption of cell-matrix communication, which is known to influence cellular differentiation as well as BM structure.[9,10]

As the cyst develops, cellular proliferation is clearly important for cyst expansion, and alterations in the processing and sorting of proteins lead to polarity changes.[10] Ultimately, developing cysts bud off from the nephron but continue to enlarge, indicating that the epithelia have changed to a secretory state. It has been suggested that apoptosis may play a major role in the destruction of the normal, non-cystic nephrons in the kidney.[11] The complexity of the changes in the ADPKD kidney has made identifying the primary defect(s) difficult by biochemical and cellular methods. Consequently, progress in recent years has resulted from identifying those molecules by the genetic method of positional cloning.

Genetic heterogeneity

Genetic linkage analysis of ADPKD families soon led to the

identification of a major locus (now designated *PKD1*) on the tip of the short arm of chromosome 16 (16p13.3).[12] Although *PKD1* accounts for the majority of families (ca 85% in the European population[13]), a significant minority were unlinked to this region, and a second locus (*PKD2*) on chromosome 4 was ultimately identified.[14,15] The presence of a small group of families unlinked to either of these loci suggests that there may be at least one more ADPKD gene.[16–18]

Clinical manifestations

The clinical manifestations of PKD1 and PKD2 are very similar, with many of the extrarenal complications frequently found in PKD1 (eg liver cysts, intracranial aneurysms) also found in PKD2 families.[19,20] There is, however, an important difference in the severity of renal disease, with PKD1 more severe than PKD2. PKD1 typically has an earlier age of clinical presentation, is more likely to be associated with hypertension and an average age of onset of ESRD about 14 years earlier than for PKD2 (60.3 years vs 74 years).[19,21] The similarities of these two disorders, though, suggest that the PKD1 and PKD2 proteins may interact or form part of the same biochemical pathway.

Cloning the autosomal dominant polycystic kidney disease genes

The PKD1 gene

Despite the linkage to chromosome 16 in 1985, the *PKD1* gene was not identified until 1994, with the aid of an unusual family segregating a chromosome 16;22 translocation[22] in which the translocation break-point was found to disrupt a gene encoding a large transcript (ca 14 kb). Its identity was confirmed with the identification of mutations of this gene in other PKD1 families.[22] This family also aided the identification of a second disease gene, one for the dominant disease tuberous sclerosis, which lies immediately next to *PKD1* in a tail-to-tail orientation.[23]

Full characterisation of the *PKD1* gene, which proved difficult, showed a transcript of 14,136 bp separated into 46 exons spread over about 52 kb of genomic DNA.[24,25] It was difficult because the 5' three-quarters of the transcript is encoded by a genomic area that is reiterated several times at a second site more proximal on chromosome 16 (16p13.1).[22] This homologous region also encodes several transcripts (the homologous gene cDNAs) that share substantial homology with *PKD1* (ca 97% sequence identity), although it is not known whether they encode functional proteins.

The PKD2 gene

The *PKD2* gene was identified in 1996 when a significant region of homology was identified between a protein encoded by a cDNA from the linkage defined target region on chromosome 4 and the PKD1 protein.[26] The PKD2 transcript of about 5.7 kb is divided into 15 exons and spread over about 68 kb of genomic DNA.[27]

The autosomal dominant polycystic kidney disease proteins

Predicted structures

PKD1 protein. The predicted PKD1 protein, polycystin 1, is large (4,302 amino acids) with a calculated unglycosylated molecular weight of about 460 kDa.[24,25] Polycystin 1 contains several regions of homology with known protein motifs, but the precise structure and function of the protein has proved difficult to determine because the combination of domains is unique. The most likely model indicates that it is attached to the cell membrane via multiple transmembrane regions with a large extracellular region and short cytoplasmic tail (Fig 1). The recognised motifs at the N-terminal end, following a signal peptide, are leucine-rich repeats, flanked by cysteine-rich amino and carboxy areas and a carbohydrate recognition domain (a C type lectin). These motifs are usually involved in protein-protein or protein-carbohydrate interactions, and suggest that this region of the protein may be involved in cell-cell or cell-matrix interactions. The bulk of the predicted extracellular part of the protein consists of 16 repeats of approximately 85 amino acid sequences with distant similarity to an immunoglobulin fold.

Recent recognition of homology to a sea urchin protein[29] and comparative analysis to the polycystin 1 sequence from the puffer fish, Fugu,[28] have led to refinement of the probable structure of the remainder of the human protein. In the extracellular juxtamembrane region an area of homology of approximately 1,000 amino acids has been noted with the receptor for egg jelly protein (REJ) located on sea urchin sperm which is thought to trigger the acrosome reaction on contact with egg jelly.[29] This event involves regulation of ion channels and suggests a similar role for polycystin 1. Analysis of hydropathy profiles and topology predictions suggests the presence of 11 transmembrane domains, the first

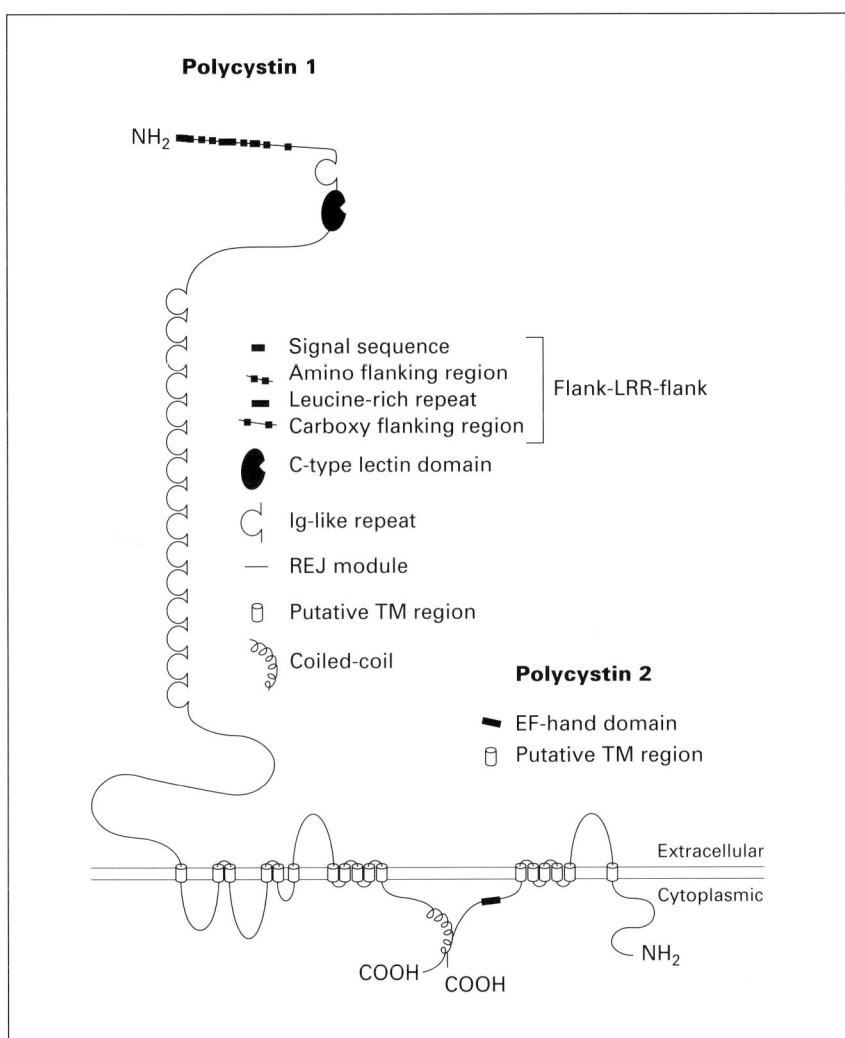

Fig 1. *Predicted models of the polycystin 1 and polycystin 2 proteins* (adapted from Refs 25, 26 and 28). Details of the characterised motifs are shown in the keys. The putative interaction between the coiled-coil of polycystin 1 and the C-terminal region of the PKD2 protein is also illustrated (COOH = carboxy end; EF hand = a specific calcium binding domain; Ig = immunoglobulin; LRR = leucine-rich repeat; NH₂ = amino end; REJ = receptor for egg jelly protein; TM = transmembrane).

matching the single domain of the REJ protein and the C-terminal 6 corresponding to those in the PKD2 protein (Fig 1).[28] The short cytoplasmic tail contains a coiled-coil domain[30] and may be involved in signalling.

PKD2 protein. The PKD2 protein is much smaller (968 amino acids), with a predicted molecular mass of about 110 kDa.[26] Polycystin 2 is also thought to be a membrane associated protein, with six transmembrane regions predicted, but in this case both N- and C- terminals are cytoplasmic (Fig 1). The region of homology with polycystin 1 extends over the entire transmembrane part of the PKD2 protein. Similarity has also been noted with the α-subunit of voltage-gated calcium and sodium channels.[26] These data, together with the REJ module in PKD1, suggest that the PKD proteins may play a role as subunits of an ion channel and/or in regulation of ion channels. A calcium-binding domain (an EF band) has also been noted in the C-terminal tail of polycystin 2.[26]

Expression

Consistent with the systemic nature of the disease, analysis of *PKD1* and *PKD2* mRNA showed expression in almost every tissue tested.[26,31] To determine the location of the proteins, antibodies to many different regions of polycystin 1 have now been described,[31-38] but no reports of polycystin 2 antibodies have yet been published. Initial studies concentrated on the expression pattern in the developing and adult kidney as the major site of disease, and some consensus is emerging from the various studies.

Polycystin is expressed in the developing kidney in the proximal regions of the ureteric bud, the maturing distal and proximal tubules, and in a region of the Bowman's capsule adjacent to the proximal tubule. Expression appears only at a low level in the nephrogenic zone of nephron induction. In the adult kidney, expression is lower and more localised to the collecting duct and distal tubules. The pattern of expression therefore reflects the sites of cyst development in ADPKD within mature tubules. Outside the kidney, fetal expression has been noted in many other epithelial structures including biliary duct, bronchial epithelia, gut lining and pancreatic ductal cells. Expression in the endothelia and smooth muscle cells of blood vessels,[39] in heart myocardium and in brain astrocytes has also been reported.[38]

The subcellular localisation of the protein is less clear, with evidence of cytoplasmic staining as well as signal on or near the basolateral and apical membranes. In one report, expression seemed to be lateral and associated with cell-cell contacts.[38] Consistent with the protein model, Western blot analysis has shown the presence of a large protein product (greater than 400 kDa) in membrane fractions.[35-37] Smaller fragments have also been seen by

Western analysis in many studies, but polycystin 1 has been demonstrated to be a particularly labile protein, and many of these fragments may be due to proteolytic degradation.[37]

One interesting finding noted in all studies is that polycystin 1 is expressed strongly in cystic epithelia from PKD1 patients. Study of tissue from a patient with a known truncating mutation of poly-cystin appears to indicate that the strong expression is not only of the abnormal protein but also from the protein generated by the normal allele.[31] This high level of expression may possibly reflect the dedifferentiated state of cystic epithelia.

Functional analysis

In an attempt to find out more about the normal role of the ADPKD proteins, much effort is being applied to identifying molecules that may interact as part of a complex or within a biochemical pathway. Initial studies have concentrated on the short cytoplasmic tail of polycystin 1, a region containing a coiled-coil domain, and *in vitro* analysis indicates that this interacts with the C-terminal region of the PKD2 protein.[30,40] The interaction appears to stabilise the PKD1 protein, with evidence also presented of homodimerisation of polycystin 2.[40] These results suggest that the ADPKD proteins may function through a common signalling pathway.

An important step to understanding the role of polycystin 1 has recently been made with the description of targeted disruption of the *PKD1* gene in the mouse.[41] A mutation has been induced within *PKD1* by removal of exon 34, resulting in a frameshifting change predicted to terminate the protein prematurely. This reflects the type of mutation seen in PKD1 patients (see later). Interestingly, no phenotype has yet been detected in the Pkd1[+/−] heterozygous mutant mouse (unlike the human dominant disease). In the Pkd1[−/−] homozygote, most animals die in late fetal life or shortly after birth with massively enlarged cystic kidneys, cystic pancreas and small hypoplastic lungs. The fetal kidneys of the Pkd1[−/−] embryos appear to develop normally for up to $14\frac{1}{2}$ days before cystic dilations appear, first in the proximal tubules of the outer medulla and later in the collecting tubules of the inner medulla and cortex. Consistent with the expression pattern of the protein, the normal development up to $14\frac{1}{2}$ days indicates that the role and action of polycystin 1 are not in the early stages of renal induction (nephrogenic condensation and epithelialisation) but in matura-tion, elongation and branching of the tubule. In one clear differ-ence from the human disease, no cysts were found in Pkd1[−/−] liver.

The reason for the lack of a phenotype in the heterozygote is not yet clear, but may reflect life expectancy and/or physiological differences between mouse and man and may provide clues about the disease mechanism (see below).

The mutation mechanism in autosomal dominant polycystic kidney disease

Mutation analysis of the *PKD1* gene has proved difficult because of the complex genomic region encoding most of the gene,[22] and most of the mutations described so far lie in the 3' single copy area or in the immediately adjacent duplicated area.[42–45] Efforts are now underway to develop methods to enable the entire gene to be screened for mutations.[46] The smaller size and lack of genomic complexity around the *PKD2* gene have made mutation screening simpler in this case.[47]

The results of the mutation analysis are similar for both loci, with a wide range of different mutations identified, most of them unique to a single family.[43,44,46,47] Thus, despite the positive family history of most ADPKD patients, it is clear that new mutations are occurring at a significant rate. With neither the *PKD1* nor the *PKD2* gene is there clear evidence of clustering of mutations, with changes found throughout the entire regions screened. Most of the described changes are stop or frameshifting changes which would be predicted to terminate the protein prematurely, and it seems likely that these are inactivating mutations.

Further evidence that mutations of *PKD1* are inactivating comes from the study of a rare group of patients who have large deletion mutations of *PKD1* which also disrupt the adjacent tuberous sclerosis gene *TSC2*.[48,49] In these cases, patients with germline changes have a phenotype of tuberous sclerosis and severe PKD, usually manifest in the first years of life. Their renal prognosis is much poorer than in typical ADPKD, with the onset of ESRD, on average, in their early 20s.[49] Detailed molecular analysis of these contiguous deletion cases revealed that a significant minority were mosaic for the mutated chromosome, and their degree of renal cystic disease was highly variable.[49] The *TSC2/PKD1* deletion patients support the notion that a null PKD1 mutation promotes cyst development because the entire *PKD1* gene is deleted in many of them. It is not clear why the disease is so severe in this situation, but may indicate that disruption of *TSC2* also has an additive cystogenic effect.

Polycystic kidney disease in the heterozygous state

If PKD1 mutations are inactivating, an important question that has generated considerable debate is why does disease occur in the heterozygous state when one normal allele is present? Recent data have suggested that *PKD1* is recessive at the cellular level and that cysts develop only when a second somatic mutation has inactivated the normal allele.[50,51] These studies have isolated cystic epithelia from single renal cysts and have shown, first, that in the majority of cases cells within the cyst are clonal[50] (suggesting a common origin) and, secondly, that loss of heterozygosity, loss of the normal allele, has occurred in approximately 25% of cysts. It is suggested that point mutations inactivate the second allele in the rest of the cysts, and one example of this has been demonstrated.[50] The idea of a second somatic event being required to initiate cystogenesis is attractive because it could explain the focal nature of the disease, in that only a small proportion of nephrons develop cysts.[7]

These results, however, appear at odds with the finding described by many groups that cystic tissue usually stains with polycystin antibodies, including evidence of staining of the protein from the normal allele.[31] These data appear reconcilable only if a high level of somatic mutation is occurring within PKD1 kidneys that allows the expression of functionally inactive protein but which is detected by immunohistology. It has been suggested that a polypyrimidine tract within intron 21 of *PKD1* may promote such mutations, but this has been studied so far only in germline cases and no clear hot spot for mutation has been highlighted.[52]

An alternative explanation may be that the somatic mutations detected in cystic tissue are not required for cyst formation but that they promote the growth or survival of a cyst. In this case, the initiation of the cyst may be due to a dosage reduction of polycystin, which could trigger a change to a cystic pathway, occurring in a stochastic way in the cells of the patient's nephrons. Further studies, especially of the *PKD1* knock-out mouse should help to resolve this uncertainty.

Conclusions

Cloning of the *PKD1* and *PKD2* genes has provided the raw material to study the primary defects in ADPKD. The role of the polycystin proteins is not yet clear, but involvement in cell-matrix and/or cell-cell interactions and associated signalling seems likely, with channel regulation and/or activity possible. Immunohistology and analysis of the Pkd2$^{-/-}$ mutant suggest a role for polycystin 1 in tubule maturation in the kidney rather than induction. Mutation analysis suggests that the ADPKD changes are inactivating, and it has been suggested that the disease may develop only after an additional somatic event. It is hoped that in the next few years a better understanding of the normal role of the ADPKD proteins and the mechanism of disease will lead to the development of an effective therapy.

Note added in proof: Targeted disruption of the mouse *Pkd2* gene has recently been described.[53] This mouse model closely resembles the human disease because cysts are seen in the *Pkd2*[+/−] heterozygous animals. In addition, cysts are more frequent in animals containing a highly mutable *Pkd2* allele, further indicating a role for somatic mutation in cyst development.

References

 1 Gabow PA, Johnson AM, Kaehny WD, Kimberling WJ, *et al.* Factors affecting the progression of renal disease in autosomal-dominant polycystic kidney disease. *Kidney International* 1992; **41**: 1311–9.
 2 Zerres K, Rudnik-Schöneborn S, Deget F. Routine examination of children at risk of autosomal dominant polycystic kidney disease. *Lancet* 1992; **339**: 1356–7.
 3 Torres VE. Polycystic liver disease. In: Watson ML, Torres VE (eds). *Polycystic kidney disease.* Oxford: Oxford University Press, 1996: 500–29.
 4 Huston J, Torres VE, Sulivan PP, Offord KP, Wiebers DO. Value of magnetic resonance angiography for detection of intracranial aneurysm in autosomal dominant polycystic kidney disease. *Journal of the American Society of Nephrology* 1993; **3**: 1871–7.
 5 Gabow PA. Autosomal dominant polycystic kidney disease – more than a renal disease. *American Journal of Kidney Disease* 1990; **16**: 403–13.
 6 Somlo S, Rutecki G, Giuffra LA, Reeders ST, *et al.* A kindred exhibiting cosegregation of an overlap connective tissue disorder and the chromosome 16 linked form of autosomal dominant polycystic kidney disease. *Journal of the American Society of Nephrology* 1993; **4**: 1371–8.
 7 Grantham JJ, Geiser JL, Evan AP. Cyst formation and growth in autosomal dominant polycystic kidney disease. *Kidney International* 1987; **31**: 1145–52.
 8 Baert L. Hereditary polycystic kidney disease (adult form): a microdissection study of two cases at an early stage of the disease. *Kidney International* 1978; **13**: 519–25.
 9 Carone FA, Bacallao R, Kanwar YS. Biology of polycystic kidney disease. *Laboratory Investigations* 1994; **70**: 437–48.
10 Carone FA, Nakamura S, Caputo M, Bacallao R, *et al.* Cell polarity in human renal cystic disease. *Laboratory Investigations* 1994; **70**: 648–55.
11 Woo D. Apoptosis and loss of renal tissue in polycystic kidney diseases. *New England Journal of Medicine* 1995; **333**: 18–25.
12 Reeders ST, Breuning MH, Davies KE, Nicholls RD, *et al.* A highly polymorphic DNA marker linked to adult polycystic kidney disease on chromosome 16. *Nature* 1985; **317**: 542–4.
13 Peters DJM, Sandkuijl LA. Genetic heterogeneity of polycystic kidney

disease in Europe. In: Breuning MH, Devoto M, Romeo G (eds). *Contributions to nephrology 97: polycystic kidney disease*. Basel: Karger, 1992: 128–39.

14   Kimberling WJ, Kumar S, Gabow PA, Kenyon JB, *et al.* Autosomal dominant polycystic kidney disease: localization of the second gene to chromosome 4q13–q23. *Genomics* 1993; **18**: 467–72.

15   Peters DJM, Spruit L, Saris JJ, Ravine D, *et al.* Chromosome 4 localization of a second gene for autosomal dominant polycystic kidney disease. *Nature Genetics* 1993; **5**: 359–62.

16   Daoust MC, Reynolds DM, Bichet DG, Somlo S. Evidence for a third genetic locus for autosomal dominant polycystic kidney disease. *Genomics* 1995; **25**: 733–6.

17   de Almeida S, de Almeida E, Peters D, Pinto JR, *et al.* Autosomal dominant polycystic kidney disease: evidence for the existence of a third locus in a Portuguese family. *Human Genetics* 1995; **96**: 83–8.

18   Bogdanova N, Dworniczak B, Dragova D, Todorov V, *et al.* Genetic heterogeneity of polycystic kidney disease in Bulgaria. *Human Genetics* 1995; **95**: 645–50.

19   Torra R, Badenas C, Darnell A, Nicolau C, *et al.* Linkage, clinical features, and prognosis of autosomal dominant polycystic kidney disease types 1 and 2. *Journal of the American Society of Nephrology* 1996; **7**: 2142–51.

20   van Dijk MA, Chang PC, Peters DJM, Breuning MH. Intracranial aneurysms in polycystic kidney disease linked to chromosome 4. *Journal of the American Society of Nephrology* 1995; **6**: 1670–3.

21   Ravine D, Walker RG, Gibson RN, Forrest SM, *et al.* Phenotype and genotype heterogeneity in autosomal dominant polycystic kidney disease. *Lancet* 1992; **340**: 1330–3.

22   European Polycystic Kidney Disease Consortium. The polycystic kidney disease 1 gene encodes a 14 kb transcript and lies within a duplicated region on chromosome 16. *Cell* 1994; **77**: 881–94.

23   European Chromosome 16 Tuberous Sclerosis Consortium. Identification and characterization of the tuberous sclerosis gene on chromosome 16. *Cell* 1993; **75**: 1305–15.

24   International Polycystic Kidney Disease Consortium. Polycystic kidney disease: the complete structure of the *PKD1* gene and its protein. *Cell* 1995; **81**: 289–98.

25   Hughes J, Ward CJ, Peral B, Aspinwall R, *et al.* The polycystic kidney disease 1 (*PKD1*) gene encodes a novel protein with multiple cell recognition domains. *Nature Genetics* 1995; **10**: 151–60.

26   Mochizuki T, Wu G, Hayashi T, Xenophontes SL, *et al. PKD2*, a gene for polycystic kidney disease that encodes an integral membrane protein. *Science* 1996; **272**: 1339–42.

27   Hayashi T, Mochizuki T, Reynolds DM, Wu G, *et al.* Characterization of the exon structure of the polycystic kidney disease 2 gene (*PKD2*). *Genomics* 1997; **44**: 131–6.

28   Sandford R, Sgotto B, Aparacio S, Brenner S, *et al.* Comparative analysis of the polycystic kidney disease 1 (*PKD1*) gene reveals an integral membrane glycoprotein with multiple evolutionary conserved domains. *Human Molecular Genetics* 1997; **6**: 1483–9.

29   Moy GW, Mendoza LM, Schulz JR, Swanson WJ, *et al.* The sea urchin

sperm receptor for egg jelly is a modular protein with extensive homology to the human polycystic kidney disease protein, PKD1. *Journal of Cell Biology* 1996; **133**: 809–17.

30 Qian F, Germino FJ, Cai Y, Zhang X, *et al. PKD1* interacts with *PKD2* through a probable coiled-coil domain. *Nature Genetics* 1997; **16**: 179–83.

31 Ward CJ, Turley H, Ong ACM, Comley M, *et al.* Polycystin, the poly-cystic kidney disease 1 protein, is expressed by epithelial cells in fetal, adult and polycystic kidney. *Proceedings of the National Academy of Sciences of the USA* 1996; **93**: 1524–8.

32 Griffin MD, Torres VE, Grande JP, Kumar R. Immunolocalization of polycystin in human tissues and cultured cells. *Proceedings of the Association of American Physicians* 1996; **108**: 185–97.

33 Peters DJM, Spruit L, Klingel R, Prins F, *et al.* Adult, fetal and poly-cystic kidney expression of polycystin, the polycystic kidney disease-1 gene product. *Laboratory Investigations* 1996; **75**: 221–30.

34 Palsson R, Sharma CP, Kim K, McLaughlin M, *et al.* Characterization and cell distribution of polycystin, the product of autosomal dominant polycystic kidney disease gene 1. *Molecular Medicine* 1996; **2**: 702–11.

35 Geng L, Segal Y, Peissel B, Deng N, *et al.* Identification and localization of polycystin, the *PKD1* gene product. *Journal of Clinical Investigation* 1996; **98**: 2674–82.

36 Geng L, Segal Y, Pavlova A, Barros EJG, *et al.* Distribution and developmentally regulated expression of murine polycystin. *American Journal of Physiology* 1997; **272**: F451–9.

37 van Adelsberg J, Chamberlain S, D'Agato V. Polycystin expression is temporally and spatially regulated during renal development. *American Journal of Physiology* 1997; **272**: F602–9.

38 lbraghimov-Beskrovnaya O, Dackowski WR, Foggensteiner L, Cole-man N, *et al.* Polycystin: *in vitro* synthesis, *in vivo* tissue expression, and subcellular localization identifies a large membrane-associated protein. *Proceedings of the National Academy of Sciences of the USA* 1997; **94**: 6397–402.

39 Griffin MD, Torres VE, Grande JP, Kumar R. Vascular expression of polycystin. *Journal of the American Society of Nephrology* 1997; **8**: 616–26.

40 Tsiokas L, Kim E, Arnould T, Sukhatme VP, Walz G. Homo- and heterodimeric interactions between the gene products of *PKD1* and *PKD2*. *Proceedings of the National Academy of Sciences of the USA* 1997; **94**: 6965–70.

41 Lu W, Peissel B, Babakhanlou H, Pavlova A, *et al.* Perinatal lethality with kidney and pancreas defects in mice with a targeted *PKDL* muta-tion. *Nature Genetics* 1997; **17**: 179–81.

42 Peral B, Gamble V, San Millán JL, Strong C, *et al.* Splicing mutations of the polycystic kidney disease 1 (*PKD1*) gene induced by intronic deletion. *Human Molecular Genetics* 1995; **4**: 569–74.

43 Peral B, Ong ACM, San Millán JL, Gamble V, *et al.* A stable, nonsense mutation associated with a case of infantile onset polycystic kidney disease 1 (*PKD1*). *Human Molecular Genetics* 1996; **5**: 539–42.

44 Peral B, San Millán JL, Ong ACM, Gamble V, *et al.* Screening the 3' region of the polycystic kidney disease 1 (*PKD1*) gene reveals six

novel mutations. *American Journal of Human Genetics* 1996; **58**: 86–96.

45   Turco AE, Rossetti S, Bresin E, Corra S, *et al*. A novel nonsense mutation in the *PKD1* gene (C3817T) is associated with autosomal dominant polycystic kidney disease (ADPKD) in a large three-generation Italian family. *Human Molecular Genetics* 1995; **4**: 1331–5.

46   Rossetti S, Ward C, Harris PC. A strategy for mutation screening in the duplicated region of the polycystic kidney disease 1 (*PKD1*) gene. *Journal of the American Society of Nephrology* 1997; **8**: 380A (abstract).

47   Veldhuisen B, Saris JJ, de Haij S, Hayashi T, *et al*. A spectrum of mutations in the second gene for autosomal dominant polycystic kidney disease (*PKD2*). *American Journal of Human Genetics* 1997; **61**: 547–55.

48   Brook-Carter PT, Peral B, Ward CJ, Thompson P, *et al*. Deletion of the *TSC2* and *PKD1* genes associated with severe infantile polycystic kidney disease – a contiguous gene syndrome. *Nature Genetics* 1994; **8**: 328–32.

49   Sampson JR, Maheshwar MM, Aspinwall R, Thompson P, *et al*. Renal cystic disease in tuberous sclerosis: the role of the polycystic kidney disease 1 gene. *American Journal of Human Genetics* 1997; **61**: 843–51.

50   Qian F, Watnick TJ, Onuchic LF, Germino GG. The molecular basis of focal cyst formation in human autosomal dominant polycystic kidney disease type 1. *Cell* 1996; **87**: 979–87.

51   Brasier JL, Henske EP. Loss of the polycystic kidney disease (*PKD1*) region of chromosome 16p13 in renal cyst cells supports a loss-of-function model for cyst pathogenesis. *Journal of Clinical Investigation* 1997; **99**: 194–9.

52   Watnick TJ, Piontek KB, Cordal TM, Weber H, *et al*. An unusual pattern of mutation in the duplicated portion of *PKD1* is revealed by use of a novel strategy for mutation detection. *Human Molecular Genetics* 1997; **6**: 1473–81.

53   Wu G, D'Agati V, Cai Y, Markowitz G, *et al*. Somatic inactivation of *Pkd2* results in polycystic kidney disease. *Cell* 1998; **93**: 177–88.

Part 3

The 1997 Teale Lecture

11 | The challenge of the meningococcus

E Richard Moxon
Department of Paediatrics; and Molecular Infectious Diseases Group, Institute of Molecular Medicine, University of Oxford

I would like first to recognise the opportunity afforded through the benefaction of Sir Francis Teale's wife, Dorothea. The endowment supports a biennial lecture on work connected with diseases of children. Sir Francis was a distinguished immunologist and microbiologist; I hope, therefore, that both Sir Francis and his wife would have approved of the title of this evening's Teale Lecture, 'The challenge of the meningococcus'. The meningococcus is the cause of devastating infections, mainly septicaemia and meningitis. These serious diseases can occur at any age, but the highest attack rates are in young infants. Thus, in this lecture dedicated to the memory of Sir Francis Teale, I am able to bring together both the emphasis on child health and his interest in microbial diseases.

The meningococcus

The meningococcus is a Gram-negative bacterium and an important feature of its biology is that it is obligately host-adapted to humans. No other natural reservoir of the organism is known and, for the most part, it colonises the human upper respiratory tract. Most individuals who become colonised with the meningococcus are, and remain, healthy so that invasive disease is a rare outcome in the context of a very common occurrence – the carrier state. The epidemiology of meningococcal carriage and disease varies with time and geographical location. In Europe and the USA, rates of invasive disease average about one case per 100,000 population per year, more than half the cases occurring in children aged less than five years. Outbreaks involving small clusters of individuals, particularly in institutions such as universities, schools or military establishments are, however, characteristic, with those involved typically young adults.

Despite antibiotics and access to sophisticated medical care (at least in our part of the world), the mortality from invasive meningococcus disease averages 10%. There is also considerable morbidity among survivors, particularly in the case of meningitis. Currently, the meningococcus is the commonest cause of acute bacterial meningitis in Europe and the USA, but this is a recent trend. Only a few years ago, cases of *Haemophilus influenzae* type b (Hib) meningitis outnumbered those of the meningococcus but, with the introduction of routine immunisation with conjugate vaccines, Hib meningitis has been virtually eliminated and the total number of all cases of bacterial meningitis halved.[1] Unlike Hib, where only one capsular serotype causes almost all episodes of invasive disease, most virulent strains of the meningococcus associated with invasive disease express one of three different polysaccharide capsules, designated serogroups A, B and C.

Epidemiology

The epidemiological importance of these different serogroups varies greatly in different countries and continents. In Europe and the USA, capsular group B strains are responsible for 50–70% of all cases and the rest by group C strains. The picture is dramatically different in sub-Saharan Africa in what has come to be known as the 'meningitis belt'.[2] Capsular group A strains account for the vast majority of invasive disease which occurs in the form of epidemics that sweep through the meningitis belt every few years. For reasons that are poorly understood, group A strains that are so devastating in causing these epidemics in Africa are extremely uncommon in Europe and the USA – indeed, even carriers of group A strains are rare.

Pathogenesis of the meningococcus

What then is known about the characteristics of the meningococcus that are responsible for its pathogenic potential? An appreciation of its virulence factors warrants a close look at the cell envelope or outer layer of the bacterium which comes into contact with the host. The main mode of action of the capsular polysaccharide as a major virulence factor of meningococci is to impede phagocytosis and complement-mediated lysis. Virulence, however, is complex. Over the past few years, many other microbial factors of the meningococcus have been identified as important contributors to its pathogenicity including pili, outer membrane proteins and lipopolysaccharide. The application of molecular genetics and cell

biology has also opened the doors to a relatively detailed understanding of the pathogenesis of invasive meningococcal infections.

Pili (fimbriae)

For example, one of the critical characteristics of any pathogenic
microbe is its ability to establish relatively stable colonisation of
host tissues. To this end, pili (sometimes referred to as fimbriae)
act as an adhesin for attaching meningococci to human cells such
as the epithelia of the respiratory tract. Pili are also responsible for
the tropism of meningococci for man, since the adhesin is specific
for receptors found on certain human cells but not other animals.[3]
Pili are filamentous structures predominantly consisting of a major
subunit polypeptide supplemented by a smaller number of minor
proteins. The subunit polypeptide is encoded by the *pilE* gene
family, a family of genes and partial gene sequences which provides
a repertoire of coding regions so that the assembled pili on any
one meningococcal bacterial cell surface is one of a large number
of possible variants.[4] Current thinking is that these variants allow
escape from host-immune responses so that the subunit acts rather
like a decoy for confusing the immune system. There is evidence
that the adherence function of pili is carried out by a minor
protein, *pilC*, which is closely associated with the major filamentous
protein made up of the subunits. There is still some controversy
about the precise nature of the interaction of pili with human
epithelial cells in the upper respiratory tract, but mutations
(either *pilE* or *pilC*) have a dramatic effect on the ability of the
meningococcus to adhere to epithelial cells.[5]

Outer membrane proteins (opacity proteins)

Pili are, however, by no means the whole story about attachment to
human cells. Indeed, one of the general features of pathogenic
bacteria in general is that there is considerable redundancy with
regard to these important host-interactive functions. The meningococcus is no exception, and another set of molecules involved in
interactions of the meningococcus with epithelial cells includes the
outer membrane proteins, the so-called opacity proteins, of which
one example is Opc.[6]

This outer membrane protein is of interest in that it not only
mediates adherence but also facilitates invasion of cells. Its
mechanism of interaction with host cells is particularly intriguing.
In contrast to the current evidence concerning pili, where a minor

protein acts as a ligand to attach to a host receptor, Opc has a more subtle strategy. It can bind to its surface host proteins, such as vitronectin and, once vitronectin is bound to Opc, the latter can mediate its attachment to host cells through the same mechanism that vitronectin uses to engage with its natural receptor, a surface integrin.[7]

The role of surface molecules of the meningococcus

These insights into pathogenesis suggest a key role for surface molecules of the meningococcus involved in promoting tropism for human cells, thereby facilitating colonisation and invasion of host tissues.

The capsule acts to inhibit clearance of organisms that have invaded the blood. This sets up the events leading to disease, and raises the issue of the identity of molecules involved in the tissue injury characteristic of meningococcal septicaemia and meningitis.

Lipopolysaccharide (LPS) is the best understood of the several candidate molecules associated with the induction of inflammation and tissue damage. LPS is a complex glycolipid in which the molecular components can be assigned very different functions. A hydrophobic component, lipid A (often referred to as endotoxin), anchors the molecule to the cell envelope of the meningococcus. Many details of the ability of lipid A to induce inflammation are yet to be understood, but it is clear that particular structural features such as fatty acylation and phosphorylation are critical to its function.[8] Although the carbohydrate portion of the molecule (inner and outer core oligosaccharides) may modulate these functions, mutants resulting in virtually complete truncation of the oligosaccharides retain the inflammatory mediating properties.

Lipid A interacts with host cells through an intricate set of mechanisms that are only recently becoming understood at the molecular level. Several binding proteins have been identified, including LPS binding protein. This complex allows interaction with either soluble or membrane-bound host CD14,[9] which results in signal transduction to release pro-inflammatory mediators such as cytokines. Not surprisingly, this interaction lies at the heart of understanding one of the major pathophysiological factors in the biology of the shock and inflammation associated with meningococcal sepsis and meningitis.

This series of complex cascades involving multiple interactions of host and microbial determinants is under intense investigation, with the hope that unravelling these events could lead to novel therapeutic approaches.

Prevention of meningococcal infections: vaccines

The rapidity with which invasive meningococcal infections progress and the short time lapse between the first symptoms and serious illness indicate that the highest priority needs to be given to prevention. Realistically, in many parts of the world, the logistics and costs of therapy and the management of established disease impose such insuperable difficulties that this approach cannot provide any reasonable prospect of reducing the enormous morbidity and mortality, particularly in large-scale epidemics. Effective vaccines, therefore, offer the best strategy for controlling the impact of meningococcal infections.

Group A and C strains

Currently, there are licensed vaccines of proven efficacy against group A and C strains, but both have serious limitations relating to their relative lack of immunogenicity and capacity to provide robust and long-lasting protection, especially following vaccination of young infants.[10] The development of conjugates seems certain to overcome many of the inadequacies of the current polysaccharide group A and C vaccines.

Group B strains

No licensed vaccine currently exists to protect against group B strains, which in Europe and the USA account for considerably more than half of all cases of invasive meningococcal disease. Research into group B meningococcal vaccines has identified major problems in using the capsular polysaccharide as a candidate immunogen. The group B polysaccharide is a homopolymer of neuraminic acid which mimics the polysialic acid (PSA) modifications of human cell surface molecules such as neural cell adhesion molecule (NCAM).[11] Not surprisingly, PSA is extremely poorly immunogenic, presumably reflecting tolerance to a self antigen. Strategies aimed at enhancing the immunogenicity of group B polysaccharides, for example through conjugation, have proved difficult and may pose insuperable problems. The induction of long-lived serum immunoglobulin G antibodies in female infants is considered to be particularly problematical. NCAM is especially prevalent on neuronal cells of developing human brain; if a woman immunised with a vaccine based on group B poly-saccharides became pregnant, there would be the potential for cross-reactive antibodies to cross the placenta and interact with fetal brain. NCAM plays an important role in neuronal migration, so antibodies to PSA could modulate brain development of the fetus and have deleterious consequences. It is therefore sensible to consider alternative strategies for preventing group B invasive disease.[12]

Candidate immunogens

Outer membrane proteins. Several groups have been investigating outer membrane proteins of the meningococcus as candidate immunogens. This research has proved promising. Vaccines based on outer membrane vesicle preparations derived from selected strains of meningococci have demonstrated in clinical trials a sufficient degree of protection to warrant continuing research.

One problem with this approach is that the outer membrane proteins which are the targets of protective immunity are prone to genetic shift and drift. Thus, it is to be expected that variations in natural populations of meningococci may include, or give rise to, strains possessing outer membrane proteins that cannot be targeted by these vaccines.[13]

Inner core lipopolysaccharide components. We have been investigating the candidacy of conserved (inner core) components of LPS of the meningococcus. There is now a considerable body of data[14–20] on the molecular details of meningococcal LPS (Fig 1), which has led to investigating the potential of serum antibodies to access inner core epitopes to protect against invasive disease. For this approach to be feasible, it must be shown that certain epitopes are absolutely conserved, that they are accessible to antibodies and that these antibodies are protective. Candidate vaccines could then be developed using defined components of LPS that have been found to be safe and immunogenic.

The concept of LPS vaccines for prevention of meningococcal infections is not new, but the technology available for pursuing the candidacy of LPS as a vaccine has changed critically over the most recent few years. Using a combination of molecular genetics and structural biology, my laboratory has been investigating:

• the extent of conservation of inner core LPS epitopes among all strains of meningococci;

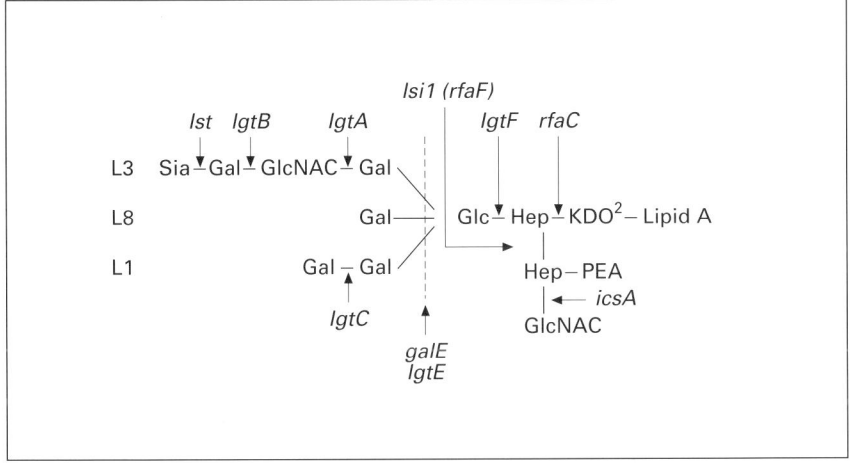

Fig 1. *A representation of the structure of meningococcal lipopolysaccharide (LPS).* The LPS molecule is depicted such that lipid A (extreme right) would be embedded in the cell envelope of the bacterial outer membrane. According to current molecular models, the terminal oligosaccharides (extreme left) are located furthest away from the bacterial cell envelope. Three distinct structural variations (immunotypes L1, L3 and L8) are shown (see related Refs 14–20). Differences between the immunotypes are indicated to the left of the vertical dotted line that marks the junction between inner (right) and outer (left) core structures. Genes for incorporating each of the key sugars or amino sugars into the LPS oligosaccharide in the biosynthetic pathway are shown by arrows indicating where in the pathway the gene product is required. Immunotype L7 LPS has a similar structure to that of L3 but lacks the terminal neuraminic acid (Gal = galactose; Glc = glucose; GlcNAC = N-acetylglucosamine; Hep = heptose; Ig = immunoglobulin; KDO = 2-keto-3-deoxyoctulosonic acid; PEA = phosphoethanolamine; Sia = N-acetylneuraminic acid).

- the accessibility of these epitopes to antibodies; and
- the functional (protective) activity of antibodies directed to these conserved and accessible LPS epitopes.

This has led to a programme of vaccine development. The approach has been facilitated by identifying the genes involved in key steps of the biosynthesis of LPS and then making a series of defined mutants. After determining their structure, these LPS mutants were used to derive monoclonal antibodies, which in turn have been used to determine how conserved and accessible are LPS epitopes of the inner core among a variety of meningococcal strains. LPS derived from inner core mutants has also been used to develop enzyme-linked immunoassays to determine the prevalence of natural antibodies in the sera of infants, children and adults.

Conclusion

Invasive diseases caused by *Neisseria meningitidis* represent a serious global public health problem. Despite many advances, the rapidity of onset and severity of meningococcal disease are such that reduction of the resulting morbidity and mortality is best achieved through immunisation. Substantial progress has been made in developing effective vaccines against serogroup A and C strains. The development of a vaccine against group B strain, the cause of more than 60% of invasive infections in the UK, remains elusive but is a high priority for current and future research.

References

1 Booy R, Heath PT, Slack MPE, Begg N, Moxon ER. Surveillance of vaccine failures following primary immunisation of infants with Hib conjugate vaccine: evidence for protection without boosting. *Lancet* 1997; **349**: 1197–202.

2 Lapeyssonnie L. La méningite cérebro-spinale en Afrique. *Bulletin of the World Health Organisation* 1963; **28**: 3–114.

3 Stephens DS, Farley MM. Pathogenic events during infection of the human nasopharynx with *Neisseria meningitidis* and *Haemophilus influenzae*. *Reviews of Infectious Diseases* 1991; **13**: 22–33.

4 Saunder JR, O'Sullivan H, Wakeman J, Sims G, *et al*. Flagella and pili as antigenically variable structures on the bacterial surfaces. *Journal of Applied Bacteriology* 1993; **74** (Suppl): 33–42.

5 Rudel M, van Putten JPM, Gibbs CP, Has R, Meyer TF. Interaction of two variable proteins (PilE and PilC) required for pilus-mediated adherence of *Neisseria gonorrhoeae* to human epithelial cells. *Molecular Microbiology* 1992; **6**: 3429–50.

6 Olyhoek AJM, Sarkari J, Bopp M, Morelli G, Achtman M. Cloning and expression in *Escherichia coli* of *opc*, the gene for an unusual class 5 outer membrane protein from *Neisseria meningitidis*. *Microbial Pathogenesis* 1991; **11**: 249–57.

7 Virji M, Makepeace K, Moxon ER. Distinct mechanisms of interactions of Opc-expressing meningococci at apical and basolateral surfaces of human endothelial cells; the role of integrins in apical interactions. *Molecular Microbiology* 1994; **14**: 173–84.

8 Lüderitz T, Brandenburg K, Seydel U, Roth A, *et al*. Structural and physicochemical requirements of endotoxins for the activation of arachidonic acid metabolism in mouse peritoneal macrophages *in vitro*. *Journal of Biochemistry* 1989; **179**: 11–6.

9 Wright SD, Tobias PS, Ulevitch RJ, Ramos RA. Lipopolysaccharide (LPS) binding protein opsonizes LPS-bearing particles for recognition by a novel receptor on macrophages. *Journal of Experimental Medicine* 1989; **170**: 1231–41.

10 Frasch CE. Meningococcal vaccines: past, present and future. In: Cartwright K (ed). *Meningococcal disease*. Chichester: John Wiley & Sons Ltd, 1995: 245–83.

11 Finne JM, Leinonen M, Mäkelä PH. Antigenic similarities between brain components and bacteria causing meningitis. Implications for vaccine development. *Lancet* 1983; **ii**: 355–7.

12 Lifely MR, Moreno C, Lindon JC. An integrated molecular and immunological approach towards a meningococcal group B vaccine. *Vaccine* 1987; **5**: 11–26.

13 Feavers IM, Fox AJ, Gray S, Jones DM, Maiden MCJ. Antigenic diversity of meningococcal outer membrane protein PorA has implications for epidemiological analysis and vaccine design. *Clinical and Diagnostic Laboratory Immunology* 1996; **3**: 444–50.

14 Jennings MP, Hood DW, Peak IRA, Virji M, Moxon ER. Molecular analysis of a locus for the biosynthesis and phase variable expression of the lacto-N-neotetraose terminal LPS structure in *Neisseria meningitidis*. *Molecular Microbiology* 1995; **18**: 729–40.

15 Gilbert M, Watson DC, Cunningham AM, Jennings MP, *et al*. Cloning of the lipooligosaccharide alpha-2,3-sialyltransferase from the bacterial pathogens *Neisseria meningitidis* and *Neisseria gonorrhoeae*. *Journal of Biological Chemistry* 1996; **271**: 28271–6.

16 Jennings MP, van der Ley P, Wilks KE, Maskell DJ, *et al*. Cloning and molecular analysis of the galE gene of *Neisseria meningitidis* and its role in lipopolysaccharide biosynthesis. *Molecular Microbiology* 1993; **10**: 361–9.

17 Kahler CM, Carlson RW, Rahman MM, Martin LE, Stephens DS. Two glycosyltransferase genes, *lgtF* and *rfaK*, constitute the lipooligosaccharide *ice* (inner core extension) biosynthesis operon of *Neisseria meningitidis*. *Journal of Bacteriology* 1996; **178**: 6677–84.

18 Jennings MP, Bisercic M, Dunn KLR, Virji M, *et al*. Cloning and molecular analysis of the *lsil* (*rfaF*) gene of *Neisseria meningitidis* which encodes a heptosyl-2-transferase involved in LPS biosynthesis: evaluation of surface exposed carbohydrates in LPS mediated toxicity for human endothelial cells. *Microbial Pathogenesis* 1995; **19**: 391–407.

19 Zhou D, Lee NG, Apicella MA. Lipopolysaccharide biosynthesis in *Neisseria gonorrhoeae*: cloning, identification and characterization of the alpha 1,5 heptosyltransferase I gene (*rfaC*). *Molecular Microbiology* 1994; **14**: 609.

20 Pavliak V, Brisson JR, Michon F, Uhrin D, Jennings HJ. Structure of the sialylated L3 lipopolysaccharide of *Neisseria meningitidis*. *Journal of Biological Chemistry* 1993; **268**: 14146–52.

Part 4

Complex multigene disorders

12 | Genetics of type 2 diabetes

Philippe Froguel
Genetics of Multifactorial Diseases, Institut de Biologie de Lille, Institut Pasteur de Lille, France

Diabetes mellitus affects about 4% and 7% of the European and US populations, respectively, and it is believed that in the next century one individual in 10 will develop diabetes. Types 1 and 2 diabetes mellitus are both multifactorial diseases, with genetic and environmental factors interacting to favour their development. Clinical and genetic heterogeneity are extreme in both types of diabetes. Although genetic and environmental factors contribute to the development of non-insulin dependent diabetes mellitus (NIDDM) and obesity, the precise molecular mechanisms leading to uncontrolled hyperglycaemia or weight gain are largely unknown. Consequently, the usual treatments often fail to induce a good glucose control that will avoid vascular complications.

Molecular mechanisms

Patients with NIDDM have defects in insulin action, abnormal insulin secretion and increased hepatic glucose production, but the precise pathways responsible for these defects have not been identified.[1]

Uncontrolled hyperglycaemia

The presence of hyperglycaemia *per se* has multiple metabolic effects on the liver, pancreatic beta cell and muscle. This clouds the primary defects, making it impossible to determine which are primarily responsible for diabetes and which result from the presence of hyperglycaemia or hyperinsulinaemia.

Obesity

Similarly, the primary causes of obesity in humans are unknown, although it is clear that both genetic and environmental factors (decreased physical activity) play a role. Despite the identification of several obesity genes in rodent models and the studies in mice lacking proteins implicated in the regulation of feeding or thermo-genesis, the key genetic and biochemical mechanisms leading to the excessive accumulation of fat mass in humans are still poorly understood.

Non-insulin dependent diabetes mellitus and obesity susceptibility genes

It is now commonly accepted that the identification of NIDDM and obesity susceptibility genes will not only allow a better understanding of the pathophysiology of diabetes but also lead to major progress in its prevention and to the provision of better care to patients.

NIDDM appears to be a heterogeneous syndrome composed of subtypes strongly associated with environmental factors at one end of the spectrum and highly genetic forms at the other.[2] Therefore, a first approach has been to differentiate the potential monogenic forms of diabetes as a paradigm for genetic studies.[3] In some respects, this strategy was successful in families showing early-onset NIDDM or severe insulin resistance, and led to the identification of mutations in several genes.

Monogenic forms of non-insulin dependent diabetes mellitus

Maturity-onset diabetes of the young (MODY), characterised by early age of onset (childhood, adolescence or young adulthood) and autosomal dominant inheritance, has been the most inten-sively investigated monogenic form of NIDDM in the last few years. Its well defined mode of inheritance, with high penetrance and early age of onset, made MODY an attractive model for genetic studies of NIDDM. It encompasses several monogenic entities:

- diabetes caused by a mutation in the hepatocyte nuclear factor 4-alpha gene (*HNF-4a/MODY1*) situated on chromosome 20q;
- diabetes caused by mutations in the glucokinase gene (*GCK/MODY2*) on chromosome 7p;
- diabetes related to mutations in the hepatocyte nuclear factor 1-alpha gene (*HNF-1a/MODY3*) situated on chromosome 12q;
- one or more other forms of diabetes still to be identified.[4-7]

More important, abnormalities in other genes encoding transcription factors may also contribute to other forms of NIDDM or their complications. In some cases, the definition of specific clinical subgroups of NIDDM may facilitate the genetic search. Indeed, in another well defined subset of diabetes associated with hearing loss, monogenic maternal inheritance has been shown to be due to a single mutation in mitochondrial DNA.[8] A few families have insulin gene mutations, and some individuals with severe insulin resistance have mutations in the insulin receptor.[9,10] However, these defects account for no more than 5% of NIDDM cases.

Identification of responsible genes

Segregation studies

The role of heredity in the common forms of type 2 diabetes is complex. It is determined by the interaction of several genes, each probably having relatively small effects, with environmental factors.[3] Segregation studies have, however, shown that familial NIDDM may be determined by major gene effects. Most of the NIDDM genes identified so far have been found through a candidate gene approach. This pathophysiological approach is not easy because maintenance of normal glucose homeostasis in the postprandial state depends on three major processes: glucose intake which stimulates insulin secretion which, in turn, promotes glucose uptake into peripheral tissues, primarily muscle and, to a lesser extent, fat tissues. Insulin also suppresses hepatic glucose output.

All three components of the system appear to be defective in NIDDM. The relative primacy of defective insulin *secretion* versus defective insulin *action* is unknown, but prospective studies of pre-NIDDM subjects indicate genetic susceptibility at the level both of cellular insulin action and of pancreatic beta cell function.[11,12] Investigation of candidate genes for NIDDM revealed a mutation in the glucagon receptor gene and the insulin receptor substrate-1 gene, and also polymorphisms in the sulfonylurea receptor gene (part of the K-channel) contributing to the genetic risk for diabetes.[13–15]

Regions of synteny

Another approach is the study of regions of synteny from polygenic animal models of NIDDM. When chromosomal regions linked with obesity or impaired glucose homoeostasis have been localised, researchers will be able to take advantage of this knowledge to examine the role that the syntenic regions may play in man.

Animal models

The study of NIDDM genetics in humans is hampered by the interference of environmental risk factors and the existence of overlapping pathophysiological features such as hypertension and obesity. This situation makes the use of inbred animal models that develop spontaneously the main features of NIDDM an important component of genetic investigations. For instance, the spontaneously diabetic Goto-Kakisaki rat strain shows the main characteristics of NIDDM and a polygenic control of diabetes-related phenotypes. Using highly polymorphic microsatellite markers spanning the 21 chromosomes of the rat genome, linkage has been demonstrated between these markers and six independently segregating quantitative trait loci predisposing to fasting hyperglycaemia, glucose intolerance or altered insulin secretion.[16]

Genome scanning

The scanning of the entire genome of NIDDM families with anonymous microsatellite markers is now performed by different groups worldwide. This method may also have limited power to dissect the loci for complex disease traits.[3] Genome screening in a relatively isolated Mexican-American diabetic population from Texas mapped a new niddm1 locus on chromosome 2, but this gene has not yet been identified. Furthermore, an NIDDM susceptibility locus was recently mapped on chromosome 20q in several Caucasian populations, and an niddm2 locus was also found on chromosome 12q near the *MODY3* gene in some insulin-deficient NIDDM families.[17–20]

Future therapy

Positional cloning and comparative gene expression studies will provide clues to understanding the molecular mechanisms of NIDDM. At this stage, the challenge is to validate targets and select the most promising for drug discovery. The potential of a gene to serve as a target for the development of new therapeutics can be evaluated either directly (the gene as the target) or indirectly (some other component in the biochemical pathway affected by the gene as the target). To do so, it will be necessary to determine the exact function of the gene and the effects on function of NIDDM or obesity-associated variants, and then to place this in an appropriate cellular and physiological context. This will be achieved by functional studies which involve complementary approaches.

References

1 De Fronzo RA. The triumvirate: beta-cell, muscle, liver: a collusion responsible for NIDDM. *Diabetes* 1988; **37**: 667-87.

2 Froguel Ph, Hager J, Vionnet N. Genetics of type 2 diabetes. *Current Opinion in Endocrinology and Diabetes* 1995; **2**: 285-9.

3 MacCarthy MI, Froguel Ph, Hitman GA. The genetics of non insulin-dependent diabetes mellitus: tools and aims. *Diabetologia* 1994; **37**: 959–68.

4 Froguel Ph, Zouali H, Vionnet N, Velho G, *et al.* Familial hyper-glycemia due to mutations in glucokinase: definition of a sub-type of diabetes mellitus. *New England Journal of Medicine* 1993; **328**: 697–702.

5 Vaxillaire M, Boccio V, Philippi A, Vigouroux C, *et al.* A gene for maturity onset diabetes of the young (MODY) maps to chromosome 12q. *Nature Genetics* 1995; **9**: 418–23.

6 Yamagata K, Furata H, Oda N, Kaisaki PJ, *et al.* Mutations in the hepatic nuclear factor 1 alpha gene in maturity-onset diabetes of the young (MODY3). *Nature* 1996; **384**: 455–8.

7 Yamagata K, *et al.* Mutations in the hepatocyte nuclear factor 4 alpha gene in maturity-onset diabetes of the young (MODY1). *Nature* 1996; **384**: 458–60.

8 Kadowaki T, Kadowaki H, Mori Y, Tobe K, *et al.* A subtype of diabetes mellitus associated with a mutation of mitochondrial DNA. *New England Journal of Medicine* 1994; **330**: 962–8.

9 Steiner DF, Tager HS, Chan SJ, Nanjo K, *et al.* Lessons learned from molecular biology of insulin-gene mutations. *Diabetes Care* 1990; **13**: 600–9.

10 Taylor SI. Molecular mechanisms of insulin resistance: lessons from patients with mutations in the insulin-receptor gene (Lilly lecture). *Diabetes* 1992; **41**: 1473–90.

11 O'Rahilly SP, Nugent Z, Rudenski AS, Hosker JP, *et al.* Beta-cell dys-function rather than insulin sensitivity is the primary defect in familial type 2 diabetes. *Lancet* 1986; **ii**: 360–4.

12 Martin BC, Warram JH, Krolewski AS, Bergman RN, *et al.* Role of glucose and insulin resistance in the development of type 2 diabetes mellitus: results of a 25-year follow-up study. *Lancet* 1992; **340**: 925–9.

13 Hager J, Hansen L, Vaisse C, Vionnet N, *et al.* A missense mutation in the glucagon receptor gene is associated with familial non-insulin dependent diabetes mellitus. *Nature Genetics* 1995; **9**: 299–304.

14 Hitman G, Hawrami K, MacCarthy MI, Viswanathan M, *et al.* Insulin receptor substrate-1 gene mutations in NIDDM: implications for the study of polygenic disease. *Diabetologia* 1995; **38**: 481–6.

15 Hani EH, Clément K, Velho G, Vionnet N, *et al.* Genetic studies of the

sulfonylurea receptor gene locus in NIDDM and obesity among French Caucasians. *Diabetes* 1997; **46**: 688-94.

16   Gauguier D, Froguel P, Parent V, Bernard C, *et al.* Chromosomal mapping of genetic loci associated with non-insulin dependent diabetes in the GK rat. *Nature Genetics* 1996; **12**: 38–43.

17   Hanis CL, Boerwinkle E, Chakraborty R, Ellsworth DL, *et al.* A genome-wide search for human NIDDM genes reveals a major susceptibility locus on chromosome 2. *Nature Genetics* 1996; **13**: 161–6.

18   Hani EH, Hager J, Philippi A, Demenais F, *et al.* Mapping NIDDM susceptibility loci in French families: studies with markers in the region of NIDDM1 on chromosome 2q. *Diabetes* 1997; **46**: 1225–6.

19   Zouali H, Hani EH, Philippi A, Vionnet N, *et al.* A susceptibility locus for early-onset non-insulin-dependent (type 2) diabetes mellitus maps to chromosome 20q, proximal to the phosphoenolpyruvate carboxykinase gene. *Human Molecular Genetics* 1997; **6**: 1401–8.

20   Mahtani MM, Widen E, Lehto M, Thomas J, *et al.* Mapping of a gene for type 2 diabetes associated with an insulin secretion defect by a genome scan in Finnish families. *Nature Genetics* 1996; **14**: 90–4.

13 | The genetics of asthma and atopy

Gavin Anderson and William Cookson
Asthma Genetics Group, Nuffield Department of Clinical Medicine,
John Radcliffe Hospital, Oxford

Asthma is a complex disease – certainly not one disease, but many – due to the interaction of an unknown number of environmental and genetic factors. The former include inhaled allergens (eg house-dust mite (HDM), cats, dogs, cockroaches), cigarette smoke (active and passive exposure), viral respiratory tract infections and atmospheric pollution. Asthma is common, affecting around 5% of adults and 10% of children.[1] In children, asthma is most often part of a syndrome of atopy characterised by the presence of allergy, asthma, seasonal rhinitis and eczema, which tends to occur in familial clusters. Atopy is characterised by immediate hypersensitivity reactions (wheal and flare to intradermal allergens), raised serum immunoglobulin (Ig) E and increased bronchial reactivity to specific inhaled allergens and other non-specific stimuli. A significant proportion of adult patients, however, do not have an atopic background. Defining the genetics of asthma will have a number of benefits, as listed in Table 1.

Mode of inheritance

The mode of inheritance of allergy and asthma has evaded description in terms of simple Mendelian genetics, but a number of pieces of research point to the presence of genetic determinants of the syndrome. The evidence for an inherited susceptibility to asthma includes segregation analysis and twin studies. Segregation analysis consistently suggests the presence of major genes underlying the syndrome, although analysis has suggested dominant, recessive, codominant and polygenic modes of inheritance for atopy and IgE

Table 1. Benefits from discovery of the genetic basis of asthma.

Increased and better understanding of the pathophysiology of asthma:
- which mechanisms are specific to asthma
- which mechanisms are shared by other inflammatory diseases

Improved classification of asthma:
- association of particular genotypes with distinct (severe or mild) clinical courses
- anticipation of response to particular treatments

Prevention of disease in susceptible infants:
- early recognition of children at genetic risk may make possible the prevention of illness by environmental manipulation or other intervention

New treatments for asthma:
- genetic discoveries will eventually lead to new pharmacological treatments

---

levels.[2-4] The twin studies demonstrate that the concordance for atopy and IgE levels is higher for monozygotic than for dizygotic twins.[5-8]

A number of studies have noted parent-of-origin effects in the inheritance of atopy. In particular, some – but not all – studies have demonstrated increased risk of atopy in children whose mother is atopic.[9-13] A maternal effect has also been noted in some of the molecular genetic studies of asthma and atopy.[14,15] The mechanism of this phenomenon remains obscure. Hypotheses include immunological interactions between mother and child, genetic imprinting and bias in the populations.

Several possible reasons may explain the deviation from simple Mendelian genetics:

- more than one gene in each individual may interact to produce the disease phenotype (polygenic inheritance);
- different genes may exist in different individuals (genetic heterogeneity); or
- interaction with the environment may lead to variable expression (penetrance).

In contrast to single gene disorders, such as cystic fibrosis or muscular dystrophy, genes predisposing to asthma do not usually contain mutations, but are most often variants of normal genes whose evolutionary advantage has become obscure in the current Western environment.

Defining the disease phenotype

The first obstacle encountered in the study of allergy and asthma genetics is to define the disease phenotype. In many investigations this has led to the use of intermediate phenotypes which allow objective measures of quantitative traits underlying the disease. These include the use of total or specific serum IgE levels, skin test reactions for hypersensitivity, and bronchial hyperresponsiveness. Reliance on symptom records or clinical diagnosis of asthma is open to a greater number of confounding factors. In addition, the method of selection (ascertainment) of the study population may introduce bias in several different ways.

Atopic asthma

Clinically, the most easily recognised and reliably defined asthma syndrome is atopic asthma. It demonstrates obvious familial clustering; for this reason, most effort towards elucidating the genetic causes of asthma has been directed at asthma in children and young adults, and at the underlying condition of atopy.

Genes causing disease may be found either by examining candidate genes or by the process known as positional cloning. Successful identification of genes predisposing to the illness, however, is likely to depend on a combination of positional cloning and candidate gene strategies.

Candidate genes

Many different kinds of genes may be involved in atopy and asthma and are therefore candidates for containing disease-causing polymorphisms. These include genes:

- predisposing in general to IgE-mediated inflammation,
- influencing the specific IgE response,
- influencing bronchial hyperresponsiveness independently of atopy, and
- influencing non-IgE mediated inflammation.

The same genes may have apparently dissimilar effects on components of the asthma phenotype under different environmental conditions, a phenomenon known as pleiotropy. Candidate genes can be assessed by defining polymorphisms within the gene, and testing these for associations with disease. At the moment, a plausible case could be made for as many as 30 different candidate genes in the aetiology of asthma, few of which have been examined in detail for polymorphism.

The high affinity immunoglobulin E receptor

Linkage of atopy, defined by IgE responses, to the chromosome 11q13 marker D11S97 was first found in 1989[16] and has been widely replicated.[17–20] Affected sib-pair analysis showed that linkage of atopy to chromosome 11 markers was to maternal alleles in many of our families.[21,22] This is likely to correspond to the maternal effect seen in clinical studies.[11,23–27] The recognition of the maternal effect allowed mapping of the atopy gene centromeric to the original D11S97 marker, and the demonstration that 60% or less of families with symptomatic atopy can be influenced by the chromosome 11 atopy gene.[14,28] This was followed by the localisation of the β chain of the high affinity receptor for IgE (FcεRI-β) to the same region, in close linkage to atopy.[17]

The first reported FcεRI-β polymorphisms were known as Leu181/Leu183 and Leu181,[29] now designated I181L/I183V and I181L. Maternal inheritance of both these variants was associated with severe atopy. There has, however, been great difficulty in detecting these variants, the structural reasons for which we are currently investigating.

A further search through the coding regions of FcεRI-β has identified a coding polymorphism in exon seven.[30] An adenine to guanine substitution changes amino acid residue 237 from glutamic acid to glycine (E237G) in the cytoplasmic tail of the protein. E237G is predicted to introduce a hydrophobicity change within the C-terminus of FcεRI-β. It is adjacent to the immunoreceptor tyrosine activation motif, and may affect the intracellular signalling capacity of FcεRI. The variant has been identified in diverse populations and is easily assayed. E237G was detected in 5.3% of an Australian general population sample, and was associated with various measures of atopy as well as bronchial reactivity to methacholine ($p = 0.0009$). The relative risk of individuals with E237G having asthma compared to subjects without the variant was 2.3. E237G did not show a parent-of-origin effect in this population. Although E237G associates with atopy and may be of functional importance, it cannot on its own or in combination with

I181L/I183V explain the strength of the chromosome 11q13 linkage. Further functional polymorphism in and around FcεRI-β therefore remains to be discovered.

Cytokine gene cluster on chromosome 5q

The region of the genome around chromosome 5q contains several molecules implicated in the pathogenesis of asthma and the control of IgE. The 5q23–31 region includes the genes coding for interleukins (IL)3, 4, 5, 9, 12b and 13, glucocorticoid receptor, and the β_2-adrenergic receptor (β_2-AR).

Interleukins. In sib-pair analysis on Amish families, Marsh and coworkers[31] showed a significant linkage between total IgE levels and several markers in this region, namely IL4R, interferon regulatory factor (IRF)1, IL9, D5S393 and D5S399, of which IL4R showed the strongest linkage when those subjects with antigen-specific responses were excluded ($p = 0.000004$).

These results were confirmed using sib-pair analysis by Meyers *et al*[32] on Dutch families who showed linkage of total IgE levels to IL9 ($p = 0.07$), D5S393, D5S436 and CSF-1R. Postma *et al*[33] reported linkage of chromosome markers with total IgE levels and bronchial hyperresponsiveness. The Dutch/American collaboration group[34,35] also suggest that two genes account for 78% of the genetic predisposition to high IgE levels. Interestingly, in these studies total IgE and bronchial reactivity were not co-inherited. In addition, Doull *et al*[36] have found significant allelic association between the 118 allele of the IL9 microsatellite and the total serum IgE.

We have presented results on linkage and allelic associations between chromosome 5q markers and atopic asthma phenotypes in 80 nuclear families from a larger general population sample.[37] Strong linkage could not be demonstrated to either total serum IgE or bronchial hyperresponsiveness ($p <0.01$), though there was a highly significant linkage to eosinophilia (D5S658, $p = 0.00091$). Significant allelic associations were demonstrated for microsatellite alleles with allele frequencies greater than 2%. The most significant results were:

- D5S1995 and total serum IgE ($p = 0.0035$),
- IL4RP1 and eosinophil count ($p = 0.0011$), and
- IL9 and bronchial hyperresponsiveness ($p = 0.00042$).

The IL association appears to be a different allele from that reported by Doull *et al*.[36]

At present, there is evidence for only one functional polymorphism in the 5q cytokine cluster, in the IL4 promoter.[38] We have investigated this polymorphism for associations with asthma and atopy phenotypes in two populations:[39]

1   In a general Caucasian population sample of 1,004 people, a weak association was detected to specific IgE to HDM (Dermatophagoides pteronyssinus) ($p = 0.013$).
2   In a case-control study in which asthmatic atopic probands were compared to unrelated age- and sex-matched non-atopic non-asthmatics, there was no significant association between the polymorphism and either total or specific IgE.

Hershey *et al*[40] have recently reported an association of atopy with a gain-of-function mutation in the α-subunit of the IL4 receptor on chromosome 16. They found an adenine to guanine substitution at nucleotide 1902, resulting in the transcription of the amino acid arginine rather than glutamine at position 576 (R576). This allele was associated with enhanced signalling of the IL4 receptor and increased CD23 expression. In a small population screened they found the R576 allele in four of seven patients with severe atopic dermatitis and in 13 of 20 subjects with atopy compared to five of 30 without atopy. This interesting result awaits confirmation in a larger population.

The β₂-adrenergic receptor. β₂-AR, which is located on chromosome 5q32, is the target for the principal class of agents (β₂-agonists) used to treat the acute bronchoconstriction in asthmatics. It is widely expressed in the lung on mast cells and bronchial smooth muscle cells. Nine point mutations have been described within the β₂-AR gene, four of which result in amino acid substitutions: Arg16→Gly, Gln27→Glu, Val34→Met and Thr164→Ile.[41] These polymorphisms were not found to be more common in asthmatics than controls. However, Gly16 was more frequent in steroid-dependent asthmatics or those who had been treated with immunotherapy. Gly16 has also been found to be more frequent than expected in asthmatics with nocturnal disease than non-nocturnal asthmatics.[42] In subsequent studies, Gly16 homozygotes were shown to have a greater loss of bronchodilator response than Arg16 homozygotes following chronic β₂-agonist treatment.[43] These associations may be explained by the increased agonist-mediated downregulation of β₂-AR demonstrated by *in vitro* studies.[44] The Glu polymorphism has been associated with reduced bronchial responsiveness.[45]

Chromosome 12q15–q24.1

The presence of the genes for interferon-γ, stem cell factor (also known as mast cell growth factor), insulin-like growth factor-1 and the β-subunit of nuclear factor-y makes this region an attractive candidate for asthma and atopy susceptibility loci. Barnes *et al*[46] have recently reported the linkage of asthma and total serum IgE concentrations on chromosome 12q in two populations: 29 Afro-Caribbean families (ascertained through 29 asthmatic probands) and 11 Amish kindreds. Linkage was detected in the Afro-Caribbean families to asthma at D12S379 (p = 0.001) and log (total serum IgE) at D12S360 (p = 0.001). The Amish population showed replication at a lower level of significance for log (total serum IgE) at D12S360 (p = 0.01). A multipoint analysis of asthma in the Afro-Caribbean families showed a peak close to D12S379 (p = 0.003).

T cell receptor-α and HLA-DR

The development of disease in atopic individuals depends on the type of allergens to which they react,[47,48] and children with HDM allergy have a greater risk of asthma than children who respond purely to grass pollen. It is therefore of clinical interest to investigate the genetic control of the specific IgE response. Inhaled allergen sources such as HDM or grass pollen are complex mixtures of proteins. For HDM, the two most important allergens are *Der p* I (25.4 kDa) and *Der p* II (14.1 kDa), each of which seems to have four major B cell epitopes.[49,50] Peptide mapping of *Der p* II has shown that T cell clones from different individuals may also react to common T cell epitopes.[51]

The HLA and T cell receptor (TCR) genes are candidates for germline influences on specific allergen responses. The association of HLA haplotypes and ragweed allergy was the first human immune response gene to be recognised,[52] and HLA-DR restriction of IgE reactions to allergen is well documented.[53,54] However, the HLA genes on their own do not account for the differences in individual IgE reactions to allergen.[20] Polymorphisms in the TCR genes influence the peripheral TCR repertoire,[55–57] and may have effects on the immune response to antigen. We have therefore examined the TCR loci for genomic restriction of IgE responses.

We have previously established linkage of specific IgE responses to the TCR-α/δ locus on chromosome 14 (but not to TCR-β) in two sets of subjects.[58] The TCR-α/δ region is complex,[59] and contains many elements which might influence specific antigen recognition. Localisation of these elements depends on associations between specific alleles and IgE responses. It was previously demonstrated that Vα8 may be in excess in T cell clones reacting to HDM,[60] and we have now investigated a bi-allelic polymorphism in Vα8.1 for association with IgE titres to HDM and its major antigens.[61] The subjects were also HLA-DR typed to investigate possible interactions between HLA and TCR loci.

In a panel of 400 subjects, allele 2 of the Vα8.1 polymorphism (Vα8.1*2) showed a significant association with higher IgE titres to *Der p* II ($p = 0.006$), and a weak association to *Der p* I ($p = 0.057$).[62] The association with Vα8.1*2 was confirmed in a second set of 400 subjects from the same population ($p = 0.03$), and was highly significant in the pooled subjects ($p = 0.001$). The IgE titres were approximately 25% higher in subjects with Vα8.1*2 in both groups and in the combined data.

Multiple regression analysis was carried out to account for possible interacting effects with HLA-DRB1, with IgE titre to *Der p* II as the dependent variable, and Vα8.1 and the six most common HLA-DR types as independent variables. Both Vα8.1*2 and HLA-DRB*1501 were shown to be positively associated with IgE titres to *Der p* II in both sets of subjects and also in the pooled data ($p = 0.0001$ for both Vα8.1 and HLA-DRB1*1501). The mean *Der p* II IgE titre in the pooled data when Vα8.1*2 and HLA-DRB1*1501 were together in the same subject was 1.14 ± 0.14 radio-allergosorbent test (RAST) classes, compared to 0.56 ± 0.025 when neither allele was present. This level of enhanced IgE response is likely to be of clinical significance.

These results indicate that germline elements in the TCR-Vα region interact with particular HLA-DR types to modify the response to foreign antigen.

Tumour necrosis factor

Airway inflammation is a prominent feature of asthma.[63,64] The pro-inflammatory cytokine tumour necrosis factor (TNF), which is prominent is asthmatic airways,[65] shows constitutional variation in the level of secretion linked to polymorphisms within the TNF gene complex and the surrounding major histocompatibility complex (MHC).[66–68] We have studied 413 subjects (92 of whom were asthmatic, as defined by questionnaire) in 88 nuclear families from a general population sample for association with asthma and TNF polymorphisms.[69] Asthma was significantly more common in subjects possessing allele 1 of the LTα *Nco*I polymorphism

(LTα *Nco*I*1) (*p* = 0.005), and allele 2 of the TNF-308 polymorphism (TNF-308*2) (*p* = 0.004). The association was confined
to the LTα *Nco*I*1/TNF-308*2 haplotype, so it was not possible to
differentiate between the effects of LTα *Nco*I and TNF-308 alleles.
The HLA-DR locus was excluded as a cause of this association.

The log$_e$ IgE did not show association with either LTα *Nco*I or
TNF-308 genotypes by analysis of variance, indicating that the
association of the TNF polymorphisms with asthma is independent
of atopy.

The results show that genotypes known to correlate with
increased TNF secretion are associated with an increased risk of
asthma, and suggest that genetic influences on inflammation are
part of the pathogenesis of the disease.

Positional cloning

Positional cloning begins with the demonstration of genetic linkage (co-inheritance) of disease and genetic markers of known
chromosomal localisation, and ends with the eventual identification and sequencing of genes from the DNA. Traditionally,
finding the gene responsible for disease required the discovery of
a biochemical or physiological abnormality leading to the
isolation of an aberrant protein which was partially sequenced.
This amino acid sequence was used to produce an oligonucleotide to screen for the expressed gene, which could then be
fully sequenced. However, in many diseases there is no known
abnormal protein, and the molecular geneticist has to resort to a
number of approaches based on statistical analysis of the cosegregation (linkage) of the disease phenotype with a region of
the genome.

The availability of closely interspersed genetic markers allows the
genome to be scanned for chromosomal regions that tend to be
shared among affected relatives and to differ between affected and
unaffected family members. Linkage may be described by a number of statistics, and thresholds have been set for recognising
'suggestive', 'significant' and 'replicated' linkages.[70,71] The most
commonly employed markers are microsatellites that contain di-,
tri-, and tetranucleotide repeats. Dense microsatellite maps with
markers at distances of 0.005–0.01% recombination are available.
Analysis of many markers in large numbers of families is made
practical by the use of highly automated genotyping using fluores-
cent-tagged oligonucleotide primers and the polymerase chain
reaction. Once a linkage is established, a number of approaches

are necessary to home in on the aberrant gene. The techniques of physical mapping have been reviewed elsewhere.[72,73]

Genome-wide search for asthma-associated traits

It is apparent that candidate loci do not account for all the genetic predisposition to asthma. To identify systematically genetic loci influencing asthma, our group has recently completed a genome-wide search for linkage to asthma-associated traits.[15] These included four quantitative parameters:

- total serum IgE,
- skin test index (STI),
- peripheral blood eosinophil count, and
- bronchial responsiveness to methacholine (slope).

A RAST index was also calculated, but gave no additional information to that from the STI. To account for pleiotropy, the categorical trait of 'atopy' was used, based on a combination of the STI, RAST index, and total serum IgE. Linkage to quantitative traits was tested by the Haseman-Elston sib-pair technique, and to atopy by affected sib-pair methods.

The prevalence of atopy in Western populations is 40–50%, and we have found that the recruitment of families with asthma in multiple members results in samples in which 70% or more subjects are atopic, with severe loss of power to detect linkage.[71] For this reason, the 80 families in the genome screen were subselected from a population sample to include non-atopic members. It was also reasoned that detection of linkage to quantitative traits would be enhanced by inclusion of subjects in normal and abnormal ranges of the trait distributions. These families contained a total of 203 offspring, forming 172 sib-pairs. The families were initially screened with 269 markers (253 autosomal and 16 X-linked).

Six regions of potential linkage ($p < 0.001$) were detected with one or more phenotypes on chromosomes 4, 6, 7, 11, 13 and 16. A Monte Carlo procedure was applied to calculate the number of false positive linkages. The Monte Carlo simulation predicted that 1.6 false-positive observations (linkages) would occur at a significant level of $p < 0.01$. As the actual number of regions of linkage observed in this study exceeds that predicted to be false positive, finding this number of loci is unlikely to have occurred by chance.

Chromosomes 11 and 16 exhibited potential linkage to IgE levels. The chromosome 11 marker FCERB, a microsatellite in FcεRI-β, also showed linkage to the STI. The regions on chromosomes 4 and 7 were linked to bronchial responsiveness, whereas the region on chromosome 6 (near the class I genes of the MHC) was linked to eosinophil counts. Weaker evidence of linkage (p <0.01) was found with other phenotypes for the markers on chromosomes 6 and 7. Markers from chromosome 13 around D13S153 showed evidence of linkage to the atopy phenotype in affected sib-pair analyses.

The markers showing p <0.001 for linkage were tested for replication in an additional panel of 77 nuclear and extended families recruited from clinics in the UK who had been used previously to map atopy on chromosome 11q13. They contained 215 offspring (268 sib-pairs), of whom 61% were atopic and 56% asthmatic (reflecting their origin through clinics).

Linkage with asthma was found to FCERB (p = 0.003) and to chromosome 16 (p = 0.03), and linkage with atopy to chromosome 13 (p = 0.003). Chromosomes 4, 11 and 16 showed significant differences in linkage between maternal and paternal alleles. Linkage to maternal meioses was seen between chromosome 4 and atopy (p <0.05) and total serum IgE (p <0.001), and between chromosome 16 and both atopy (p <0.01) and asthma (p <0.001). As already observed,[6] FCERB showed strong maternal linkage to atopy, but there was also a strong linkage to asthma (p <0.00001) not previously noted. The finding of maternal effects at several loci favours immunological interactions between mother and child rather than genetic imprinting or anticipation as a cause of these phenomena.

Thus, Monte Carlo simulations and the replication of positive results in a second set of subjects suggest that regions of true linkage have been identified by our study.

The collaborative study on the genetics of asthma

Using a different definition of the asthma phenotype, a separate study has been reported in several ethnic groups by the American Collaborative Study on the Genetics of Asthma.[74] The following linkage was demonstrated in sib-pairs:

- Caucasian: to chromosomes 5q23–31, 6p21.3–23, 11p15, 12q14–24.2, 13q21.3, 14q11.2–13 and 19q13;
- Afro-American: to chromosomes 5p15 and 17p11.1–q11.2; and
- Hispanic: to chromosomes 2q33, 12q14–24.2 and 21q21.

The level of significance of linkage used (p <0.01) implies that some will have been false positive linkages.

Overall results from the genetic studies

Taken together, these studies demonstrate many possible new loci linked to asthma and allergy traits, although only a small number of these loci have been found to have replicated in different studies (chromosomes 5q, 6p, 11q, 12q and 13q). The discrepancies in the loci detected in the various studies, both candidate gene and genome-wide surveys, may result from genetic heterogeneity or pleiotropy. Another possibility is insufficient statistical power due to inadequate population size and/or a small individual contribution of the gene to disease phenotype producing false positive and negative linkages.[70,75,76]

The characterisation of the genes from all the loci found by the Oxford genome survey and those identified by other groups remains a formidable task requiring several years of intense effort. The story of the elucidation of the genetic basis of type I diabetes mellitus gives a direct indication of the resources required to determine the contribution of individual loci.[77] Nevertheless, progress is being made.

Conclusion

The study of the genetics and the cellular mechanisms involved in asthma and allergy will lead to greater insight into their aetiology and pathogenesis. It is hoped that much of this knowledge will prove to have practical clinical value, that it will perhaps shed light on the apparent rise in the prevalence of asthma, and explain why certain environmental factors precipitate disease in some but not all individuals exposed. The identification of relevant polymorphisms in individual children may permit prediction of the risk of developing asthma and allow disease prevention strategies to be more accurately directed. The presence of certain polymorphisms may prove useful in predicting the clinical course, its severity and response to therapy. Ultimately, genetics may result in the development of novel pharmacological and immunological treatment strategies in asthma and allergy.

References

1 Strachan DP, Anderson HR, Limb ES, O'Neill A, Wells N. A national survey of asthma prevalence, severity, and treatment in Great Britain. *Archives of Disease in Childhood* 1994; **70**: 174–8.

2 Gerrard JW, Rao DC, Morton NE. A genetic study of immunoglobulin E. *American Journal of Human Genetics* 1978; **30**: 46–58.

3　Borecki I, Rao DC, Lalouel JM, McGue L, Gerrard JW. Demonstration of a common major gene with pleiotropic effects on immunoglobulin E levels and allergy. *Genetic Epidemiology* 1985; **2**: 327–38.

4　Dizier MH, Hill M, James A, Faux J, *et al.* Detection of a recessive major gene for high IgE levels acting independently of specific responses to allergens. *Genetic Epidemiology* 1995; **12**: 93–105.

5　Edfors-Lubs M. Allergy in 7,000 twin pairs. *Acta Allergologica* 1971; **26**: 249–85.

6　Hanson B, McGue M, Roitman-Johnson B, Segal NL, *et al.* Atopic disease and immunoglobulin E in twins reared apart and together. *American Journal of Human Genetics* 1997; **48**: 873–9.

7　Marsh DG, Meyers DA, Bias WB. The epidemiology and genetics of atopic allergy. *New England Journal of Medicine* 1981; **305**: 1551–9.

8　Sandford A, Weir T, Paré P. The genetics of asthma. *American Journal of Respiratory and Critical Care Medicine* 1996; **153**: 1749–65.

9　Moffat MF, Cookson WOCM. Maternal effects in atopic disease. *Clinical and Experimental Allergy* 1998; **28** (Suppl 1): 56–62.

10　Sears MR, Holdaway MD, Flannery EM, Herbison GP, Silva PA. Parental and neonatal risk factors for atopy, airway hyper-responsiveness, and asthma. *Archives of Disease in Childhood* 1996; **75**: 392–8.

11　Kuehr J, Karmaus W, Forster J, Frischer T, *et al.* Sensitisation to four common inhalant allergens within 302 nuclear families. *Clinical and Experimental Allergy* 1993; **23**: 600–5.

12　Magnusson CG. Cord serum IgE in relation to family history and as a predictor of atopic disease in early infancy. *Allergy* 1988; **43**: 241–51.

13　Aberg N. Familial occurrence of atopic disease – not genes only. *Allergy* 1992; **47**: 81.

14　Cookson WOCM, Young RP, Sandford AJ, Moffatt MF, *et al.* Maternal inheritance of atopic IgE responses on chromosome 11q. *Lancet* 1992; **340**: 381–4.

15　Daniels SE, Bhattacharya S, James A, Leaves NI, *et al.* A genome-wide search for quantitative trait loci underlying asthma. *Nature* 1996; **383**: 247–50.

16　Cookson WOCM, Sharp PA, Faux JA, Hopkin JM. Linkage between immunoglobulin E responses underlying asthma and rhinitis and chromosome 11q. *Lancet* 1989; **i**: 1292–5.

17　Young RP, Lynch J, Sharp PA, Faux JA, *et al.* Confirmation of genetic linkage between atopic IgE responses and chromosome 11q13. *Journal of Medical Genetics* 1992; **29**: 236–8.

18　Collée JM, ten Kate LP, de Vries HG, Kliphuis JW, *et al.* Allele sharing on chromosome 11q13 in sibs with asthma and atopy. *Lancet* 1993; **342**: 936.

19　Shirakawa T, Morimoto K, Hashimoto T, Furuyama J, *et al.* Linkage between severe atopy and chromosome 11q in Japanese families. *Clinical Genetics* 1994; **46**: 228–32.

20　van Herwerden L, Harrap SB, Wong ZYH, Abramson MJ, *et al.* Linkage of high-affinity IgE receptor gene with bronchial hyperreactivity, even in absence of atopy. *Lancet* 1995; **346**: 1262–5.

21　Moffatt MF, Sharp PA, Faux JA, Young RP, *et al.* Factors confounding genetic linkage between atopy and chromosome 11q. *Clinical and Experimental Allergy* 1992; **22**: 1046–51.

22   Cookson WOCM, Young RP, Sandford AJ, Moffatt MF, *et al.* Maternal inheritance of atopic IgE responsiveness on chromosome 11q. *Lancet* 1992; **340**: 381–4.

23   Bray GW. The hereditary factor in hypersensitivity anaphylaxis and allergy. *Journal of Allergy* 1931; **II**: 205–24.

24   Magnusson CG. Cord serum IgE in relation to family history and as predictor of atopic disease in early infancy. *Allergy* 1988; **43**: 241–51.

25   Arshad SH, Matthews S, Grant C, Hide DW. Effect of allergen avoidance on development of allergic disorders in infancy. *Lancet* 1992; **339**: 1493–7.

26   Åberg N. Familial occurrence of atopic disease: genetic versus environmental factors. *Clinical and Experimental Allergy* 1994; **23**: 829–34.

27   Halonen M, Stern D, Taussig LM, Wright A, *et al.* The predictive relationship between serum IgE levels at birth and subsequent incidences of lower respiratory illnesses and eczema in infants. *American Review of Respiratory Diseases* 1992; **146**: 866–70.

28   Sandford AJ, Shirakawa T, Moffatt MF, Daniels SE, *et al.* Localisation of atopy and the β subunit of the high affinity IgE receptor (FceRI) on chromosome 11q. *Lancet* 1993; **341**: 332–4.

29   Shirakawa TS, Li A, Dubowitz M, Dekker JW, *et al.* Association between atopy and variants of the β subunit of the high-affinity immunoglobulin E receptor. *Nature Genetics* 1994; **7**: 125–9.

30   Hill MR, Cookson WOCM. A new variant of the β subunit of the high-affinity receptor for immunoglobulin E (FceRl-b E237G): associations with measures of atopy and bronchial hyper-responsiveness. *Human Molecular Genetics* 1996; **5**: 959–62.

31   Marsh DG, Neely JD, Breazeale DR, Ghosh B, *et al.* Linkage analysis of IL-4 and other chromosome 5q31.1 markers and total serum IgE concentrations. *Science* 1994; **264**: 1152–6.

32   Meyers DA, Postma DS, Panhuysen CIM, Xu J, *et al.* Evidence for a locus regulating total serum IgE levels mapping to chromosome 5. *Genomics* 1994; **23**: 464–70.

33   Postma DS, Bleeker ER, Amelung PJ, Holroyd KJ, *et al.* Genetic susceptibility to asthma-bronchial hyperresponsiveness coinherited with a major gene for atopy. *New England Journal of Medicine* 1995; **333**: 894–900.

34   Amelung PJ, Bleeker ER, Postma DS, Panhuysen CIM, *et al.* A locus regulating bronchial responsiveness maps to 5q. *American Journal of Respiratory and Critical Care Medicine* 1995; **151**: A341.

35   Panhuysen CIM, Xu J, Amelung PA, Holroyd KJ, *et al.* Evidence for two loci regulating total IgE levels. *American Journal of Respiratory and Critical Care Medicine* 1995; **151**: A341.

36   Doull IJ, Lawrence S, Watson M, Begishvili T, *et al.* Allelic association of gene markers on chromosomes 5q and 11q with atopy and bronchial responsiveness. *American Journal of Respiratory and Critical Care Medicine* 1996; **153**: 1280–4.

37   Walley AJ, Cookson WOCM. Linkage and allelic association of chromosome 5 microsatellite markers with atopic asthma phenotypes in a general population sample. *American Journal of Respiratory and Critical Care Medicine* 1997; **155**: A257.

38 Rosenwasser LJ, Klemm DJ, Dresback JK, Inamura H, *et al.* Promoter polymorphisms in the chromosome 5 gene cluster in asthma and atopy. *Clinical and Experimental Allergy* 1995; **25** (Suppl 2): 74–8.

39 Walley AJ, Cookson WOCM. Investigation of an interleukin 4 promoter polymorphism for associations with asthma and atopy. *Journal of Medical Genetics* 1996; **33**: 689–92.

40 Hershey CK, Friedrich MF, Esswein LA, Thomas ML, Chatila TA. The association of atopy with a gain-of-function mutation in the alpha sub-unit of the interleukin-4 receptor. *New England Journal of Medicine* 1997; **337**: 1720–5.

41 Reihsaus E, Innis M, MacIntyre N, Liggett SB. Mutations in the gene encoding the β_2-adrenergic receptor in normal and asthmatic subjects. *American Journal of Respiratory Cell Molecular Biology* 1993; **8**: 334–9.

42 Turki J, Pak J, Green SA, Martin RJ, Liggett SB. Genetic poly-morphisms of the β_2-adrenergic receptor in nocturnal and non-nocturnal asthma. *Journal of Clinical Investigation* 1995; **95**: 1635–41.

43 Holgate ST. Asthma genetics: waiting to inhale. *Nature Genetics* 1997; **15**: 227–9.

44 Green SA, Turki J, Innis M, Liggett SB. Amino-terminal polymorphisms of the human β_2-adrenergic receptor impart distinct agonist-promoted regulatory properties. *Biochemistry* 1994; **33**: 9414–9.

45 Hall IP, Wheatley A, Wilding P, Liggett SB. Association of Glu27 β_2-adrenoceptor polymorphism with lower airway reactivity in asthmatic subjects. *Lancet* 1995; **345**: 1213–4.

46 Barnes KC, Neely JD, Duffy DL, Freidhoff LR, *et al.* Linkage of asthma and total serum IgE concentration to markers on chromosome 12q: evidence from Afro-Caribbean and Caucasian populations. *Genomics* 1996; **37**: 41–50.

47 Sears MR, Herbison GP, Holdaway MD, Hewitt CJ, *et al.* The relative risks of sensitivity to grass pollen, house dust mite and cat dander in the development of childhood asthma. *Clinical Allergy* 1989; **18**: 419–24.

48 Cookson WOCM, De Klerk NH, Ryan GR, James AL, Musk AW. Relative risks of bronchial hyper-responsiveness associated with skin-prick test responses to common antigens in young adults. *Clinical and Experimental Allergy* 1991; **21**: 473–9.

49 Lind P, Hansen OC, Horn N. The binding of mouse hybridoma and human IgE antibodies to the major faecal allergen, *Der p I*, of Dermatophagoides pteronyssinus. *Journal of Immunology* 1988; **140**: 4256–62.

50 Chapman MD, Heymann PW, Platts-Mills TA. Epitope mapping of two major inhalant allergens, *Der p I* and *Der f I*, from mites of the genus Dermatophagoides. *Journal of Immunology* 1987; **139**: 1479–84.

51 O'Hehir RE, Verhoef A, Panagiotopoulou E, Keswani S, *et al.* Analysis of human T cell responses to the group II allergen of Dermatophagoides species: localisation of major antigenic sites. *Journal of Allergy and Clinical Immunology* 1993; **92**: 105–13.

52 Levine BB, Stember RH, Fontino M. Ragweed hayfever: genetic control and linkage to HL-A haplotypes. *Science* 1972; **178**: 1201–3.

53 Marsh DG, Meyers DA, Bias WB. The epidemiology and genetics of atopic allergy. *New England Journal of Medicine* 1981; **305**: 1551–9.

54 Young RP, Dekker JW, Wordsworth BP, Schou C, *et al.* HLA-DR and HLA-DP genotypes and immunoglobulin E responses to common major allergens. *Clinical and Experimental Allergy* 1994; **24**: 431–9.

55 Loveridge JA, Rosenberg WMC, Kirkwood TBL, Bell JI. The genetic contribution to human T-cell receptor repertoire. *Immunology* 1991; **74**: 246–50.

56 Moss PAH, Rosenberg WMC, Zintzaras E, Bell JI. Characterisation of the human T cell receptor α-chain repertoire and demonstration of a genetic influence on Vα usage. *European Journal of Immunology* 1993; **23**: 1153–9.

57 Gulwani-Akolkar B, Posnett DN, Janson CH, Grunewald J, *et al.* T cell receptor V-segment frequencies in peripheral blood T cells correlate with human leukocyte antigen type. *Journal of Experimental Medicine* 1991; **174**: 1139–46.

58 Moffatt MF, Hill MR, Cornélis F, Schou C, *et al.* Genetic linkage of T-cell receptor α/δ complex to specific IgE responses. *Lancet* 1994; **343**: 1597–600.

59 Arden B, Clark SP, Kabelitz D, Mak TW. Human T-cell receptor variable gene segment families. *Immunogenetics* 1995; **42**: 455–500.

60 Wedderburn LR, O'Hehir RE, Hewitt CRA, Lamb JR, Owen MJ. In vivo clonal dominance and limited T-cell receptor usage in human CD4+ T-cell recognition of house dust mite allergens. *Proceedings of the National Academy of Sciences of the USA* 1993; **90**: 8214–8.

61 Cornélis F, Pile K, Loveridge J, Moss P, *et al.* Systematic study of human ab T cell receptor V segments shows allelic variations resulting in a large number of distinct T cell receptor haplotypes. *European Journal of Immunology* 1993; **23**: 1277–83.

62 Moffatt MF, Schou C, Faux J, Cookson WOCM. Germline TCR-α restriction of immunoglobulin E responses to allergen. *Immunogenetics* 1997; **46**: 226–30.

63 Fraser RS, Paré JAP, Fraser RG, Paré PD (eds). *Synopsis of diseases of the chest.* Philadelphia, PA: WB Saunders Company, 1994: 635–53.

64 Djukanovic R, Roche WR, Wilson JW, Beasley CR, *et al.* Mucosal inflammation in asthma. *American Review of Respiratory Diseases* 1990; **142**: 434–57.

65 Broide DH, Lotz M, Cuomo AJ, Coburn DA, *et al.* Cytokines in symptomatic asthma airways. *Journal of Allergy and Clinical Immunology* 1992; **89**: 958–67.

66 Jacob CO, Fronek Z, Lewis GD, Koo M, *et al.* Heritable major histocompatibility complex class II-associated differences in production of tumor necrosis factor a: relevance to genetic predisposition to systemic lupus erythematosus. *Proceedings of the National Academy of Sciences of the USA* 1990; **87**: 1233–7.

67 Messer G, Spengler U, Jung MC, Honold G, *et al.* Polymorphic structure of the tumor necrosis factor (TNF) locus: an *NcoI* polymorphism in the first intron of the human TNF-β gene correlates with a variant amino acid in position 26 and a reduced level of TNF-b production. *Journal of Experimental Medicine* 1991; **173**: 209–19.

68 Wilson AG, Symons JA, McDowell TL, di Giovine FS, Duff GW. Effects of a tumour necrosis factor (TNFa) promoter base transition on transcriptional activity. *British Journal of Rheumatology* 1994; **33**: 89 (abstract).

69 Moffatt MF, Cookson WOCM. Tumour necrosis factor haplotypes and asthma. *Human Molecular Genetics* 1997; **6**: 551–4.

70 Lander ES, Kruglyak L. Genetic dissection of complex traits: guidelines for interpreting and reporting linkage results. *Nature Genetics* 1995; **11**: 241–7.

71 Thomson G. Identifying complex disease genes: progress and paradigms. *Nature Genetics* 1994; **8**: 108–10.

72 Morrison JFJ, Markham AF. PCR-based approaches to human genome mapping. PCR2: a practical approach. In: McPherson MJ, Hames BD, Taylor GR (eds). *PCR: A Practical Approach.* Oxford: Oxford University Press, 1995: 165–95.

73 Levitt RC. Molecular genetic methods for mapping disease genes. *American Journal of Respiratory and Critical Care Medicine* 1994; **150**: S94–9.

74 The Collaborative Study on the Genetics of Asthma (CSCA). A genome-wide search for asthma susceptibility loci in ethnically diverse populations. *Nature Genetics* 1997; **15**: 389–92.

75 Weeks DE, Lathrop GM. Polygenic disease: methods for mapping complex disease traits. *Trends in Genetics* 1995; **11**: 513–8.

76 Lander ES, Schork NJ. Genetic dissection of complex traits. *Science* 1994; **265**: 2037–48.

77 Todd JA, Farrall M. Panning for gold: genome-wide scanning for linkage in type 1 diabetes. *Human Molecular Genetics* 1996; **5**: 1443–8.

14 | Approaches to genetic studies of attention deficit hyperactivity disorder

Philip Asherson
Social Genetic and Developmental Psychiatry Research Centre, Institute of Psychiatry, London

Sarah Curran
Department of Academic Child Psychiatry, Institute of Psychiatry, London

Diagnosis of hyperactivity

The triad of inattentiveness, overactivity and impulsivity is recognised as a disorder in children when these behaviours are severe, developmentally inappropriate and cause impaired functioning at home and school.[1] Hyperactivity is a major cause of child behavioural problems, with significant impairments in family and social relationships and in the ability to succeed at school. The long-term outcome is poor,[2] with increased risk of social isolation and persistent psychopathology in adolescence and adulthood affecting up to 60% of cases.[3,4] There are currently two main descriptive labels for the disorder: attention deficit hyperactivity disorder (ADHD) and hyperkinetic disorder (HD). In this chapter, the term 'hyperactivity' will be used to cover both definitions.

Diagnostic criteria are given in the Diagnostic and Statistical Manual (DSM) for ADHD and in the International Classification of Diseases (ICD) for HD. Both diagnoses are based on clinical history and behavioural observation; as yet, there are no useful diagnostic tests using psychometric, neurophysiological or neuro-anatomical measures. Differences in the diagnostic criteria for hyperactivity have led to considerable confusion both in the clinical setting and in the interpretation of research findings. For example, it has become clear more recently that the marked differences in prevalence rates reported between the USA and the UK are due to the definitions used rather than to any real variation in the rates of the disorder. Defining the disorder in the different ways gives the following prevalence rates in children:

- the presence or absence of inattentive, hyperactive or impulsive behaviour at a single time-point: 17%;
- the DSM IIIR definition: 5%;
- the more restricted ICD 10 definition: 1.5%.

Despite differences in definition, highly reliable clinical measurement and subsequent diagnosis can be obtained by trained raters using systematic methods of case history documentation, standardised rating scales and structured interviews. In addition, there is now a great deal of agreement between the latest ICD 10 and DSM IV definitions, which both list the same set of symptoms for inattention, hyperactivity and impulsivity. Although ADHD and HD are categorical diagnoses, they correlate highly with extreme scores on dimensional scales measuring individual variation in attention and impulsivity. The relationship between problems of attention and overactivity in the general child population and in children with an ADHD/HD diagnosis is not yet clear, and for research purposes both dimensional and categorical approaches are appropriate.[5]

A major complication in the diagnostic process is the high level of comorbidity with other childhood psychiatric disorders. Comorbidity is an important factor in determining the likely outcome and management of an individual. In the USA, as many as two-thirds of elementary school children with ADHD referred for clinical evaluation have at least one other diagnosable psychiatric disorder.[6–8] The major comorbid conditions include disorders of:

- language and communication,
- learning,
- conduct and oppositional defiance,
- anxiety,
- mood, and
- Tourette's syndrome.[7]

Genetic aetiology

The precise aetiology of hyperactivity remains unknown. It is likely that the diagnostic criteria encompass a heterogeneous group of disorders with a complex interaction of overlapping and non-overlapping aetiological factors. However, the importance of genetic factors on the concurrent manifestation of inattentiveness, impulsivity and overactivity has been clearly demonstrated using classical genetic approaches. Together with the rapid advances in gene mapping technology, this has persuaded many researchers that it is now feasible to characterise the susceptibility genes involved.

Most research so far on the genetic basis of hyperactivity addresses the familiality and heritability of the disorder. Traditional methods of behavioural genetic analysis using family, twin and adoption studies have recently been enhanced by biometric model-fitting, and there is now a widespread interest in identifying the separate and interactive effects of genetic and environmental factors.[9,10]

Family studies

Early family studies were fraught with methodological problems, such as reliance on retrospective diagnosis, clinical variability in proband diagnosis and the absence of blind case-control designs. These studies found that ADHD is approximately five times more frequent in the relatives of ADHD probands than in the general population. In addition, relatives were observed to have higher rates of conduct, oppositional, anxiety and affective disorders.[11–15]

More recent studies have introduced methodological refinements. For example, psychiatric control groups have been used[16–18] and comorbidity assessed.[18–20] These studies, which used the broad DSM III and DSM IIIR criteria rather than the more restrictive DSM IV or ICD 10 criteria, support the earlier findings. They obtained consistent evidence of a high incidence of ADHD among first-degree family members of male[21,22] and female[23,24] ADHD probands and cases presenting in adulthood.[25] Szatmari *et al*[26] found evidence of family clustering of attentional problems in a general population-based sample, suggesting that familial aggregation of these disorders is not confined only to clinic cases.

Given the considerable comorbidity in ADHD, it is possible that it might be familial when it is secondary to a comorbid condition. For example, Biederman *et al*[27] suggest that ADHD comorbid with conduct disorder may represent a distinct subtype. This suggestion is, however, contradicted by data from twin studies which show that overlap between ADHD and conduct disorder in young children with an early age of onset is due to common genetic variance.[28,29] On the other hand, Silberg *et al*[29] showed that in older children with a later age of onset (10–16 years) at least some of the genetic effects appear to be specific to the two behaviours. One interpretation of these findings is that conduct disorder is an epiphenomenon of ADHD in the younger age group, whereas comorbidity in the older group reflects a different set of genes emerging to account for conduct symptoms in adolescence.

Biederman *et al*[27] also conclude that ADHD comorbid with anxiety disorder is genetically distinct from other forms of ADHD. However, data from Plizka *et al*[30] suggest that ADHD and anxiety are distinct disorders, with different levels of overactivity and response to stimulants. Twin data from Gilger *et al*[31] show that, while in general ADHD and reading disability are distinct, a comorbid subtype may exist. In support of this, Stevenson *et al*[32] found that most of the observed variance between hyperactivity and spelling problems is due to common genetic factors. Faraone *et al*[33] found that comorbidity of ADHD with mood disorders, especially bipolar affective disorder, may reflect yet another subtype of ADHD. Evidence for genetic links between ADHD and Tourette's syndrome has also been reported in some studies,[34] but not supported by others.[35,36]

Twin studies

Twin studies have invariably shown that ADHD and related phenotypes are highly heritable, and provide compelling evidence for the importance of genetic factors. They also show that genetic factors are important for the expression of dimensional traits of behaviour related to hyperactivity, such as *normal* levels of activity,[37,38] scores of impulsivity,[39] and aspects of temperament such as activity, vigour, impulsiveness and sociability.[40]

Goodman and Stevenson[41] studied a large general population sample of 570 13 year old twins using rating scales for hyperactivity. They included multiple informants to ascertain whether the hyperactivity was situational or pervasive. The estimated heritability for clinically significant inattention and hyperactivity was 0.64. Thapar *et al*,[42] who examined a population sample of 287 8–16 year old twins, derived a dimensional score of hyperactivity from maternal ratings and estimated heritability to be in the order of 0.88. In a larger study, Levy *et al*[43] studied a sample of 2,350 twins from the Australian National Health and Medical Research Council Twin Registry using a maternal rating scale. The results suggested that DSM IIIR ADHD is highly heritable (0.92 ± 0.7). Similar findings came from reports by Gjone *et al*[44] using a general population sample and Gillis *et al*[45] using a subset of twin pairs participating in the Colorado Reading Project.[46]

Separation/adoption studies

Twin research can lead to overestimates of the effects of genetic factors in situations in which environmental factors contribute substantially to the manifestation of the trait. However, confirmatory evidence for the heritability of ADHD has been provided by adoption studies that afford better control for environmental variation (eg sibling interaction, sibship size). The basic assumption is that the frequency of a disorder which has a genetic basis should be greater among biological relatives than adoptive relatives. Data from two early studies reported higher rates of hyperactivity in biological parents of probands than in the adoptive parents.[11,47] However, both studies relied on retrospective recall of hyperactive symptoms and failed to study the biological parents of the adopted hyperactive children. Van den Oord *et al*[48] studied biologically related and unrelated sibling pairs of international adoptees (111 pairs and 221 pairs, respectively) and a group of adoptees (94) who grew up as singletons. In this study, two groups of children, hyperactive and controls, were raised by adoptive parents. An estimated 47% of the variance in parental ratings of attention was explained by genetic factors, with no significant sibling interaction or shared environmental effects.

Mode of inheritance

The number of genes influencing hyperactivity and the size of their effect remain unknown. Some authors have proposed that single genes may account for familial aggregation of the disorder,[49] but this is unlikely. Findings from other complex (non-mendelising) genetic disorders such as Alzheimer's disease, non-insulin dependent diabetes and breast cancer, show that single genes may account for the disorder in some families, but these are rare events and explain only a very small proportion of affected cases. In behavioural disorders such as schizophrenia and autism, extensive linkage studies have failed to identify genes of major effect and it is clear that a few or – perhaps more likely – many genes are involved.

In hyperactivity, the expected size of effects from individual gene loci can be gauged by consideration of the ratio of the risk for the disorder in first-degree relatives of probands compared to the general population risk (ca 5). The low relative risk means that if a single locus is found to explain all the genetic risk for the disorder, the genotypic relative risk (risk conferred by the risk genotype to population risk) itself could equal no more than five. It is, however, more probable that a few or many genes are involved, so the genotypic risks for individual loci are likely to be in the order of two or less. This size of gene effect has clear implications for the approaches to be taken in identifying susceptibility genes in hyperactivity.

Linkage strategies

Positional cloning

To date, great progress has been made in mapping disease genes for disorders with known single gene inheritance using positional cloning. Once suitable families have been ascertained, it has become relatively simple to scan the genome for linkage between a chromosomal region and the disorder using a coarse map of markers at 10 cM intervals. The entire genome is approximately 3,500 cM long, so 350 markers are sufficient for comprehensive scans for linkage. When a linkage region has been found, individual families can be studied in more detail to identify key recombinants which define markers flanking the disease gene. The aim is to define the target region to a physical distance of no more than 2 Mbp. The '2 Mbp problem' can then be resolved by forming a series of overlapping clones, known as a contig, which contain the full DNA sequence of the target region. Genes within the contig can then be identified and screened for functional mutations associated with the disorder.

The positional cloning approach has proved successful in the study of complex genetic disorders, where rare genetic subtypes with clear single gene inheritance have been identified. However, genes identified in this way have not in general been shown to confer susceptibility to the common forms of these disorders. The problem with this approach to linkage, which uses the logarithm of the odds score method of analysis, is the requirement to specify the genetic parameters of gene penetrance and frequency. The method therefore lacks power in the face of genetic and aetiological heterogeneity. These parameters are unknown for hyperactivity, and the large multiply affected families needed for this type of analysis are likely to contain multiple disease genes.[50,51]

Allele sharing

More promise in mapping susceptibility genes in complex disorders has been shown with allele sharing methods of linkage analysis. Most studies have adopted an affected sibling pairs strategy based upon large collections of nuclear families (parents plus affected sibling pairs). These families are relatively easy to collect and more representative of the disorder than larger multiplex families. A non-parametric statistic is derived by comparing the number of alleles shared at a particular locus between affected siblings with the number of shared alleles expected under random segregation. Excess sharing of a chromosomal region suggests linkage and the localisation of a susceptibility gene. The first major study of this type was in type 1 diabetes, and was highly successful in identifying at least five different susceptibility loci.[52] This approach has been far less successful in schizophrenia and manic depression,[53] asthma[54,55] and multiple sclerosis,[56] although recent results in juvenile myoclonic epilepsy[57] and autism[58] look promising. The problem is the power of allele sharing methods to detect genes of small effect, rather than moderate effect, in realistic sample sizes of affected sibling pairs.[59]

Association strategies

An alternative strategy is to look for disease-gene associations in general populations. This type of approach has far more power to detect genes of small effect in realistic sample sizes and is set to become an even more powerful tool as the Human Genome Project progresses. Association studies are performed by looking for allele frequency differences between samples of unrelated probands and of controls. Control genotypes can come from a series of unaffected individuals representative of the population from which the proband sample is drawn or by using the non-transmitted alleles of the proband's parents.

There are several reasons for association between a disorder and an allele. First, the association may be due to tight linkage between the allele being tested and a susceptibility locus. This can occur only when the two loci are very close together. For most human populations, appreciable allelic associations are likely to exist only for loci with recombination fractions of 1% or less (<1 cM).[60] For a large, random mating population, the relationship between the distance between two loci and magnitude of association is described by the equation: $k = \log(0.5)/\log(1-\theta)$, where k is the number of generations to halve the magnitude of association and θ is the recombination fraction. For example, it takes 693 generations to halve the magnitude of association between two loci 0.1 cM apart, 69 generations if they are 1 cM apart and 6.5 generations if they are 10 cM apart.

A second interesting cause for association is pleiotropy. Here, the genetic polymorphism is a functionally significant variant (FSV), and is itself the cause of disease susceptibility.

A less interesting cause of allelic association is population stratification where the case and control samples are derived from different populations in which alleles occur at different frequencies. In addition, mere chance differences may occur between case and control samples. The problem of population stratification can be overcome by the use of parental genotypes as controls. In the haplotype relative risk analysis[61] of parent-proband trios, the alleles transmitted to the proband become the case genotypes, whereas the non-transmitted alleles become the control genotypes.

Another useful approach using trios is the transmission disequilibrium test[62] which is a test for both linkage and association.

To date, association strategies in complex disorders have focused on targeting candidate genes and candidate regions. Genes are targeted where there is an *a priori* hypothesis for their involvement in a disorder. Associations between the gene and the disorder of interest are looked for using either nearby anonymous polymorphic markers or FSVs within the gene. The search for FSVs in genes of interest has intensified in recent years, since associations will be much stronger for markers within the gene which must lie very close to putative pathological variants or may be pathological variants themselves. However, for disorders like hyperactivity in children, we have little idea what constitutes a likely candidate. Over 80% of all genes are expressed within the central nervous system, and we are aware of the functional significance of only a tiny proportion of them. It is therefore likely that in the future a far more profitable strategy will be to screen the entire genome for association.[63]

Association versus linkage: power considerations

The power of affected sibling pair linkage versus that of association has been compared by Risch and Merikangas.[59] These authors argue that linkage approaches have limited power to detect genes of small effect in complex disorders, and that association studies have far greater power when testing all loci in the genome. They illustrate the power of linkage versus association for different genotypic relative risks by determining the sample size N necessary to obtain 80% power (Table 1). Assuming that the susceptibility allele occurs reasonably frequently (eg APOE4 occurs on 10% of chromosomes in Alzheimer's disease), the power of association is such that samples of 1,000–2,000 individuals will detect genotypic relative risks as low as 1.5.

Table 1. The number of families needed to identify a disease gene with 80% power at $\alpha = 5 \times 10^{-8}$ (this assumes that all possible loci are examined in a genome-wide scan) (adapted from Ref 59).

Genotypic relative risk	Frequency of disease allele	Linkage (no. of sib-pairs)	Association (no. of singletons)
4.0	0.01	4,260	1,098
	0.10	185	150
	0.50	297	103
	0.80	2,013	222
2.0	0.01	296,710	5,823
	0.10	5,382	695
	0.50	2,498	340
	0.80	11,917	640
1.5	0.01	4,620,807	19,320
	0.10	67,816	2,218
	0.50	17,997	949
	0.80	67,816	1,663

Candidate gene studies in hyperactivity

Studies on candidate genes have already started, with several groups examining genes involved in dopaminergic neurotransmission due to the well characterised clinical response of hyperactivity to stimulants. Dopamine transporter (DAT) 1 is particularly interesting since it is the primary site of action of methylphenidate whose main action is to inhibit the transporter.[64] Mice lacking DAT1 have been shown to display marked spontaneous hyperlocomotion because of the persistence of dopamine in the synaptic cleft.[65] The first report on a haplotype relative risk study between a variable number of tandem repeat polymorphisms at the DAT1 locus and DSM IIIR-diagnosed ADHD and undifferentiated attention deficit disorder found significant evidence of an association (n = 49, $p = 0.006$).[66] Two later studies obtained similar results with DAT1,[67,68] although other studies have failed to replicate them.[69,70]

La Hoste *et al*[71] report a significant association between the variable 48 bp repeat found within the dopamine D4 receptor gene and ADHD. These data have been further extended by Sunohara *et al*[72] who found an increased frequency of the 7-repeat – of particular interest since this variant has previously been shown to mediate a blunted intracellular response to dopamine.[73] Furthermore, the 7-repeat has been reported to be in association with the personality trait of novelty-seeking.[74,75] Further studies in ADHD samples support these initial findings,[76] although others fail to replicate them.[67,77]

Possible explanations for discrepant results

Conflicting reports of this type are not uncommon in the psychiatric genetic literature. There are several possible explanations, which will need to be addressed before it can confidently be stated whether one or both of these genes are true susceptibility loci for ADHD:

1 The samples collected by different centres vary due to variation in local clinical practice, the method of clinical assessment and diagnostic criteria. These differences may have a marked effect on the phenotype being studied. For example, Cook *et al*[66] used the DSM IIIR definition of ADHD which allows comorbidity with other psychiatric diagnoses. This may not be important for those with comorbid conduct disorder, which is likely to be a complication of hyperactivity, but those with comorbid anxiety or depression may have an entirely distinct condition.
2 In all the studies to date, the sample sizes have been small (40–100) and lack the power either to exclude or to replicate the reported associations.
3 The levels of significance reported are high, given the low *a priori* odds of detecting a true association, so that mere chance alone remains a feasible explanation.

It is clear that progress in this field will be better served by independent groups adopting a common set of diagnostic measures and clinical criteria. This will facilitate the analysis of large, clinically consistent samples by either pooling clinical data sets or performing meaningful meta-analyses. A collaborative network has recently been set up to achieve this in the UK and Ireland.

Identification of candidate loci with animal models

Animal models of hyperactivity may also identify candidate loci. A recent report describes a mouse model of hyperkinesis which implicates a gene, *Snap-25*, in behavioural regulation.[78] The mouse mutant coloboma (Cm/+) exhibits profound spontaneous locomotor hyperactivity which is due to a large deletion spanning several genes, including *Snap-25*. Administration of amphetamine markedly reduces locomotor activity, paralleling the clinical effect of dopamine agonists in hyperactivity. When a transgene encoding *Snap-25* was bred into the coloboma strain, the mice exhibited normal levels of locomotor activity. The gene is known to play an important role in the vesicular release of neurotransmitters into the synapse, including monoamines such as dopamine. Further work is now required to identify FSVs from the human homologue of this gene and to test them for associations in appropriate clinical samples.

Mapping of genes responsible for animal model behaviours

Another approach is to map genes which account for model behaviours in animals. The Wistar-Kyoto and Wistar-Kyoto hyperactive rat strains are known for their low and high activity levels, respectively. Moisan *et al*[79] reported the detection of a major quantitative trait locus (QTL) on chromosome 8, which explains 29% of the genetic variance between the behaviours of these two strains. This chromosomal region is represented by syntenic regions (homologous segments of chromosome containing similar genes) on mouse chromosome 9 and sections of human chromosomes 11q, 15q and 3p. It is possible that the human homologue of the rat QTL may influence hyperactivity in children, and attempts now need to be made to identify the gene in rat (and hence in human) and/or map around the syntenic human chromosomal regions.

Genome scans for association

Genome scans for association have not yet been performed because up to now the number of genotypes which would need to be generated has been prohibitively large. As described above, association between two adjacent loci in most large populations is unlikely to extend beyond 1 cM. Since the genome is approximately 3,500 cM long, a dense map of at least 3,500 markers would be required. Modern genotyping equipment has revolutionised the rate of genotyping, and the 350 markers needed for a linkage study can now be performed in 200 individuals in about four months in most academic laboratories – and much quicker where equipment and staff resources are more plentiful. However, the task of typing ten times this number of markers in total sample sizes of at least 400 remains too daunting both in time and cost.

DNA pooling

Over the last year there has been a great deal of interest in approaches in which individual DNA samples are pooled, a technique known as DNA pooling.[80,81] It has been successfully used to map linkage regions in autosomal recessive disorders using genetically isolated populations, but has yet to be applied to association studies of complex disorders. The method is best suited to a case-control design in which only two pools are required: pools of all the case samples and of all the control samples. It is easy to see the dramatic effect a pooling approach would have on the number of genotypes: for a sample of 200 cases and 200 controls, only 7,000 (2 × 3,500) genotypes would need to be performed in an initial screen, compared to 1,400,000 genotypes using conventional methods.

The technique is not however without its difficulties, which stem mainly from the properties of the polymerase chain reaction and microsatellite markers (simple sequence repeat polymorphisms). At present, the only available marker maps for this type of high density screening consist mainly of dinucleotide repeats.[82] The peak patterns displayed by these markers show additional artefactual bands due to slippage of the Taq enzyme on the repeat part of the template and the differential amplification of small allele fragments over long ones. This makes it impossible simply to read off the relative peak heights and estimate with any accuracy the true allele frequencies within the pool of DNA.

There are ways round this problem, such as forming a mathematical matrix for each marker,[80] but this greatly increases the time needed to set up the system. Alternatively, it is possible simply to look for differences in the crude allele patterns.[81] In either case, the method can be greatly enhanced by taking a multiphase approach to study design, which provides a balance between false positives and false negatives in the search for susceptibility genes.[80] For example, in phase I, 200 cases and controls are screened for all 3,500 markers. The top 10% of markers (350) showing differences between case and control pools are then screened in an independent phase II sample, with the top 10% of markers (35) from that sample used for an analysis of probands and their parents to protect against possible ethnic stratification effects.

Future approaches

The future holds even more promise that all the susceptibility genes for hyperactivity in childhood and related disorders will be identified. An improved marker map is currently being developed which will contain around 10,000 single base-pair substitutions.[83,84] These polymorphisms are frequent within the genome, occurring on average every 500–1,000 bp. New methods to genotype these markers are also being developed, using a technique of allele specific hybridisation to very dense arrays of oligonucleotides attached to physical supports such as glass or silicon chips.[85] In addition, there is the prospect that by the year 2006 there will be sequence available for the entire human genome. It should then be possible to identify both the location of most genes and the polymorphic variation for all the genes in the human genome, and perhaps also to perform the ultimate mapping experiments – that is, to screen large and well characterised clinical samples for associations using functionally significant variants from all human genes.[63]

References

1   Swanson JM, Sergeant JH, Taylor E, Sonuga-Barke E, *et al.* Attention-deficit hyperactivity disorder and hyperkinetic disorder. *Lancet* 1998; **351**: 429–33.

2   Taylor E. Dysfunctions of attention. In: Cicchetti D, Cohen DJ (eds). *Developmental psychopathology*, vol 2. New York: Wiley Press, 1995: 243–73.

3   Barkley RA. Attention-deficit/hyperactivity disorder. In: Mash EJ, Barkley RA (eds). *Child psychopathology*. New York: Guilford Press, 1996: 63–112.

4   Hill JC, Schoener EP. Age dependent decline of ADHD. *American Journal of Psychiatry* 1996; **153**: 1143–6.

5   Taylor E. Similarities and differences in DSM IV and ICD 10 diagnostic criteria. In: Greenhill LL (ed). *Child and adolescent clinics of North America*, vol 3. No. 2. *Disruptive disorders*. Philadelphia, PA: WB Saunders Company, 1994: 209–26.

6   Arnold LE, Jensen PS. Attention deficit disorders. In: Kaplan H, Sadock B (eds). *Comprehensive textbook of psychiatry*, 6th edn. Baltimore, MD: Williams & Wilkins, 1995: 2295–310.

7   Cantwell DP. *Therapeutic management of attention deficit disorder: participant workbook*. New York: SCP Communication, 1994: 4–20.

8   Nottleman E, Jensen P. Comorbidity of disorders in children and adolescents: developmental perspectives. *Advances in clinical child psychology*, vol 17. New York: Plenum, 1995: 109–55.

9   Rutter M, *et al.* Genetic factors in child psychiatric disorders. II. Empirical findings. *Journal of Child Psychology and Psychiatry* 1990; **31**: 39–83.

10 Simonoff E, McGuffin P, Gottesman II, *et al.* Genetic influences on normal and abnormal development. In: Rutter M, Taylor E, Hersov L (eds). *Child and adolescent psychiatry – modern approaches*, 3rd edn. Oxford: Blackwell Scientific Publications, 1994: 129–51.

11 Morrison JR, Stewart MA. A family study of the hyperactive child syndrome. *Biological Psychiatry* 1971; **3**: 189–95.

12 Cantwell DP. Psychiatric illness in the families of hyperactive children. *Archives of General Psychiatry* 1972; **27**: 414–7.

13 Welner Z, Welner A, Stewart M, Parkes H, Wish E. A controlled study of siblings of hyperactive children. *Journal of Nervous and Mental Diseases* 1977; **165**: 110–7.

14 Pauls DL, *et al.* Demonstration of vertical transmission of ADD. *Annals of Neurology* 1983; **14**: 363.

15 Biederman J, Munir K, Knee D, Habelow W, *et al.* A family study of patients with attention deficit disorder and normal controls. *Journal of Psychiatric Research* 1986; **20**: 263–74.

16 Biederman J, Faraone SV, Keenan K, Knee D, Tsuang MT. Family genetic and psychosocial risk factors in DSM III diagnosed ADD. *Journal of the American Academy of Child and Adolescent Psychiatry* 1990; **29**: 526–33.

17 Faraone SV, Biederman J, Keenan K, Tsuang MT. Separation of DSM III ADD and conduct disorder: evidence from a family-genetic study of American psychiatric patients. *Psychological Medicine* 1991; **21**: 109–21.

18 Perrin S, Last C. Relationships between ADHD and anxiety in boys: results from a family study. *Journal of the American Academy of Child and Adolescent Psychiatry* 1996; **35**: 988–96.

19 Biederman J, Faraone SV, Keenan K, Steingard R, Tsuang MT. Familial association between attention deficit disorder and anxiety disorders. *American Journal of Psychiatry* 1991; **148**: 251–6.

20 Biederman J, Faraone SV, Keenan K, Tsuang MT. Evidence of familial association between attention deficit disorder and major affective disorders. *Archives of General Psychiatry* 1991; **48**: 633–41.

21 Huzdiak JJ. Familial subtyping ADHD. *Current Opinion in Psychiatry* 1993; **6**: 489–93.

22 Lombroso PJ. Genetic mechanisms in childhood psychiatric disorders. *Journal of the American Academy of Child and Adolescent Psychiatry* 1994; **33**: 921–38.

23 Faraone SV, Biederman J, Keenan K, Tsuang MT. A family genetic study of girls with DSM III ADD. *American Journal of Psychiatry* 1991; **148**: 112–7.

24 Faraone SV, Biederman J, Chen WJ, Milberger S, *et al.* Genetic heterogeneity in ADHD: gender, psychiatric comorbidity and maternal ADHD. *Journal of Abnormal Child Psychology* 1995; **104**: 334–45.

25 Biederman J, Faraone S, Keenan K, Benjamin J, *et al.* Further evidence for family-genetic risk factors in attention-deficit hyperactivity disorder – patterns of comorbidity in probands and relatives in psychiatrically and paediatrically referred samples. *Archives of General Psychiatry* 1992; **49**: 728–38.

26 Szatmari P. The epidemiology of ADHD. In: Weiss G (ed). *Child and adolescent psychiatric clinics of North America.* Philadelphia, PA: WB Saunders Company, 1992: 361–72.

27 Biederman J, Newcorn J, Sprich S. Comorbidity of ADHD with conduct, depressive anxiety and other disorders. *American Journal of Psychiatry* 1991; **148**: 564–77.

28 Levy F, Hay DA, McStephen M, Wood C, Waldman I. Attention-deficit

hyperactivity disorder: a category or continuum? Genetic analysis of a large-scale twin study. *Journal of the American Academy of Child and Adolescent Psychiatry* 1997; **36**: 737–44.

29 Silberg J, Rutter M, Meyer J, Maes H, *et al.* Genetic and environmental influences on the covariation between hyperactivity and conduct disturbance in juvenile twins. *Journal of Child Psychology and Psychiatry* 1996; **37**: 803–16.

30 Plizka SR. Comorbidity of ADHD and overanxious disorder. *Journal of the American Academy of Child and Adolescent Psychiatry* 1992; **31**: 197–203.

31 Gilger JW, Pennington BF, DeFries JC. A twin study of the etiology of comorbidity: ADHD and dyslexia. *Journal of the American Academy of Child and Adolescent Psychiatry* 1992; **31**: 343–8.

32 Stevenson J, Pennington BF, Gilger JW, DeFries JC, Grillis JJ. Hyperactivity and spelling disability; testing for shared genetic aetiology. *Journal of Child Psychology and Psychiatry* 1993; **34**: 1137–52.

33 Faraone S, Biederman J, Mennin D, Russell D. Bipolar and antisocial disorders among relations of ADHD children: parsing familial subtypes of illness. *American Journal of Medical Genetics* 1998; **81**: 108–16.

34 Comings DE. The role of genetic factors in conduct disorder based on studies of Tourette's syndrome and ADHD probands and their relatives. *Developmental Behavioural Paediatrics* 1995; **16**: 142–57.

35 Pauls DL, Hurst CR, Kruger SD, Leckman JF, *et al.* Gilles de la Tourette's syndrome and ADD with hyperactivity. *Archives of General Psychiatry* 1986; **43**: 1177.

36 Pauls DL, *et al.* Familial relationships between Gilles de la Tourette's syndrome, ADD, learning disabilities, speech disorders and stuttering. *Journal of the American Academy of Child and Adolescent Psychiatry* 1993; **32**: 1044–50.

37 Scarr S. Genetic factors in activity motivation. *Child Development* 1966; **37**: 663–72.

38 Willerman L. Activity level and hyperactivity in twins. *Child Development* 1973; **44**: 288–93.

39 Gottesman II. Heritability of personality: a demonstration. *Psychological Monographs* 1963; **77**: 572.

40 Vandenberg SG. The heredity abilities study: heredity components in a psychological test battery. *American Journal of Human Genetics* 1962; **2**: 220–37.

41 Goodman R, Stevenson J. A twin study of hyperactivity. II. The aetiological role of genes. Family relationships and perinatal adversity. *Journal of Child Psychology and Psychiatry* 1989; **30**: 691–709.

42 Thapar A, Hervas A, McGruffin P. Childhood hyperactivity scores are highly heritable and show sibling competition effects: twin study evidence. *Behaviour Genetics* 1995; **25**: 537–44.

43 Levy F, Hay D, McClaughlin M, Wood C, Waldman I. Twin-sibling differences in parental reports of ADHD, speech, reading and behaviour problems. *Journal of Child Psychology and Psychiatry* 1996; **37**: 569–78.

44 Gjone M, *et al.* Genetic influence on parent-reported attention related problems in a Norwegian general population twin sample. *Journal of the American Academy of Child and Adolescent Psychiatry* 1996; **35**: 588–96.

45 Gillis JJ, Gilger JW, Pennington BF, DeFries JC. Attention deficit disorder in reading disabled twins: evidence for a genetic aetiology. *Journal of Abnormal Child Psychology* 1992; **20**: 303–15.

46 De Fries J, Fulker D. Multiple regression analysis of twin data. *Behaviour Genetics* 1985; **15**: 467–73.

47 Cantwell D. Genetic studies on hyperactive children. Psychiatric illness in biologic and adoptive parents. In: Fieve R, Rosenthal D, Brill H (eds). *Genetic research in psychiatry*. Baltimore, MD: Johns Hopkins Press, 1975.

48 Van den Oord E, Boomsma DI, Verhulst FC. A study of problem behaviours in 10–15 year old biologically related and unrelated international adoptees. *Behaviour Genetics* 1994; **24**: 193–205.

49 Faraone SV, Biederman J, Chen W, Krifcher B, *et al*. Segregation analysis of attention deficit hyperactivity disorder. *Psychiatric Genetics* 1992; **2**: 257–75.

50 Durner M, Greenberg DA, Hodge SE. Inter and intrafamilial heterogeneity: effective sampling strategies and comparison analysis of methods. *American Journal of Human Genetics* 1992; **51**: 859–70.

51 Owen MJ, Craddock N. Modern molecular genetic approaches to complex traits: implications for psychiatric disorders. *Molecular Psychiatry* 1996; **1**: 21–6.

52 Davies JL, Kawaguchi Y, Bennett ST, Copeman JB, *et al*. A genome-wide search for human type I diabetes susceptibility genes. *Nature* 1994; **371**: 130–6.

53 Moldin S. The maddening hunt for madness genes. *Nature Genetics* 1997; **17**: 127–8.

54 Holgate ST. Asthma genetics: waiting to exhale. *Nature Genetics* 1997; **15**: 227–9.

55 The Collaborative Study on the Genetics of Asthma (CSGA). A genome-wide search for asthma susceptibility loci in ethnically diverse populations. *Nature Genetics* 1997; **15**: 389–92.

56 Multiple Sclerosis Genetics Group. A complete genomic screen for multiple sclerosis underscores a role for the major histocompatibility complex. *Nature Genetics* 1996; **13**: 469–71.

57 Elmslie FV, Rees M, Williamson MP, Kerr M, *et al*. Genetic mapping of a major susceptibility locus for juvenile myoclonic epilepsy on chromosome 15q. *Human Molecular Genetics* 1997; **6**: 1329–34.

58 Maestrini E and the International Autism Consortium. A genome-wide search for autism susceptibility genes. *American Journal of Medical Genetics (Neuropsychiatric Genetics)* 1997; **74**: 567 (abstract).

59 Risch N, Merikangas K. The future of genetic studies of complex human diseases. *Science* 1996; **273**: 1516–7.

60 Sham P. The analysis of allelic association. *Statistics in human genetics*. New York: John Wiley and Sons Inc, 1998: 145–85.

61 Falk CT, Rubenstein P. Haplotype relative risks: an easy reliable way to construct a proper control sample for risk calculations. *Annals of Human Genetics* 1987; **51**: 227–33.

62 Spielman RS, McGinnis R, Ewens W. Transmission test for linkage disequilibrium: the insulin gene region and insulin-dependent diabetes mellitus (IDDM). *American Journal of Human Genetics* 1993; **56**: 777–87.

63 Collins FS. Variations on a theme: cataloging human DNA sequence variation. *Science* 1997; **278**: 158–81.

64 McCracken J. A two part model of stimulant action on attention deficit hyperactivity in children. *Journal of Neuropsychiatry* 1991; **3**: 201–9.

65 Giros B, Jaber M, Jones SR, Wrightman RM, Caron MG. Hyperlocomotion and indifference to cocaine and amphetamine in mice lacking the dopamine transporter. *Nature* 1996; **379**: 606–12.

66 Cook EH Jr, Stein MA, Krasowski MD, Cox NJ, *et al.* Association of attention deficit disorder and the dopamine transporter gene. *American Journal of Human Genetics* 1995; **56**: 993–8.

67 Gill M, Daly G, Heron S, Hawi Z, Fitzgerald M. Confirmation of association between ADHD and a dopamine transporter polymorphism. *Molecular Psychiatry* 1997; **2**: 311–3.

68 Waldman ID, *et al.* Association of the dopamine transporter gene (DAT1) and ADHD in children. *American Journal of Human Genetics* 1996; **59** (Suppl): A25.

69 Asherson P, Curran S, Simanoff E, Taylor E. Candidate gene studies in attention deficit hyperactivity disorder. *American Journal of Medical Genetics (Neuropsychiatric Genetics)* 1997; **74**: 631 (abstract).

70 Palmer C, Bailey J, Ramsey C, Cantwell D, *et al. American Journal of Medical Genetics (Neuropsychiatric Genetics)* 1997; **74**: 630 (abstract)

71 La Hoste GJ, *et al.* Dopamine D4 receptor gene polymorphism is associated with ADHD. *Molecular Psychiatry* 1996; **1**: 121–4.

72 Sunohara G, *et al.* Association of dopamine receptor gene attention deficit hyperactivity disorder. *American Journal of Human Genetics* 1996; **59**: A238 (abstract).

73 Van Tol HH, Bunzow JR, Guan HC, Sunahara RK, *et al.* Cloning of the gene for a human dopamine D4 receptor with high affinity for the antipsychotic clozapine. *Nature* 1991; **350**: 610–4.

74 Ebstein RP, Novick O, Umansky R, Priel B, *et al.* Dopamine D4 receptor (D4DR) exon III polymorphism associated with the human personality trait of novelty seeking. *Nature Genetics* 1996; **12**: 78–80.

75 Benjamin J, Li L, Patterson C, Greenberg BD, *et al.* Population and familial association between D4 dopamine receptor gene and measures of novelty seeking. *Nature Genetics* 1996; **12**: 81–4.

76 Bailey J, Palmer C, Ramsey C, Cantwell D, *et al.* DRD4 gene and susceptibility to attention deficit hyperactivity disorder: differences in familial and sporadic cases. *American Journal of Medical Genetics (Neuropsychiatric Genetics)* 1997; **74**: 622 (abstract).

77 Castellanos F, Lau E, Tayebi N, Lee P, *et al.* Evidence that a D4DR*7R dopamine receptor polymorphism is not correlated with attention deficit hyperactivity disorder. *American Journal of Medical Genetics (Neuropsychiatric Genetics)* 1997; **74**: 623 (abstract).

78 Hess E, Collins KA, Wilson MC. Mouse model of hyperkinesis implicates SNAP-25 in behavioral regulation. *Journal of Neuroscience* 1996; **16**: 3104–11.

79 Moisan MP, Couvoisier H, Bihoreau MT, Gauguier D, *et al.* A major quantitative trait locus influences hyperactivity in the WKHA rat. *Nature Genetics* 1996; **14**: 471–3.

80 Barcellos L, Klitz W, Field LL, Tobias R, *et al.* Association mapping of

disease loci, by use of a pooled DNA genomic screen. *American Journal of Human Genetics* 1997; **61**: 734–47.

81 Daniels J, Holmans P, Williams N, Turic D, *et al.* A simple method for analyzing microsatellite allele image patterns generated from DNA pools and its application to allelic association studies. *American Journal of Human Genetics* 1998; **62**: 1189–97.

82 Dib C, Faure S, Fizames C, Samson D, *et al.* A comprehensive genetic map of the human genome based on 5,264 microsatellites. *Nature* 1996; **380**: 152–4.

83 Wang D, *et al.* Toward a third generation genetic map of the human genome based on biallelic polymorphisms. *American Journal of Human Genetics* 1996; **59**: A3.

84 Kruglyal L. The use of a genetic map of biallelic markers in linkage studies. *Nature Genetics* 1997; **17**: 21–4.

85 Castellino AM. When the chips are down. *Genome Research* 1997; **7**: 943–6.

15 | Epilepsy

Frances V Elmslie
Institute of Child Health, London

Epilepsy is a term describing a heterogeneous group of conditions with a variety of aetiologies. The epilepsies have been classified according to two major criteria.[1,2] The first separates the epilepsies according to whether the seizures are generalised or partial; the second separates epilepsies of known aetiology (symptomatic) from those thought to be symptomatic but in which the aetiology is unknown (cryptogenic) and those in which there is no underlying cause other than an inherited predisposition (idiopathic).

A genetic contribution to the aetiology of epilepsy has been recognised for centuries and has been substantiated by numerous family and twin studies. In a study of 466 patients with epilepsy of all kinds, Tsuboi and Christian[3] found that 9.9% of the relatives of probands had seizures. In twin studies, the incidence of epilepsy in monozygotic (MZ) and dizygotic (DZ) twins is compared. For all epilepsy, the concordance rate is about 60% and 13% for MZ and DZ pairs, respectively. However, for individuals with specific seizure types and normal brains, the concordance rate in MZ twins seems to be even higher.[4]

Epilepsy forms part of the phenotype of over 100 Mendelian disorders including a variety of neurological and metabolic conditions. A few rare epilepsies are inherited in a Mendelian manner but the majority are inherited in a complex non-Mendelian fashion. Loci for a number of the Mendelian epilepsies have been mapped, and the genes are gradually being identified. Those for the complex phenotypes have proved more elusive, and the results obtained in a number of studies have been the subject of considerable debate.

Mendelian epilepsies

Benign familial neonatal convulsions

Benign familial neonatal convulsions (BFNC) is a rare form of idiopathic epilepsy inherited in an autosomal dominant fashion, characterised by the onset of seizures in the first few days of life, with remission occurring commonly by six weeks. The seizures are usually brief and generalised. Subsequent neurodevelopment is normal, although about 10% of individuals will develop epilepsy later.

A gene for BFNC was localised by linkage analysis to the long arm of chromosome 20 in a single three-generation family in 1989 and the locus designated *EBN1*.[5] An additional study of two North American families suggested the presence of both clinical and genetic heterogeneity.[6] Subsequently, a second locus (*EBN2*) was mapped to chromosome 8q.[7] Both genes have recently been identified.[8,9] They encode novel voltage-gated potassium channels, *KCNQ2* (*EBN1*) and *KCNQ3* (*EBN2*). These genes are members of the recently identified KQT-like class of potassium channels, the only previously identified member of which is *KCNQ1* (*KVQT1*) (the gene mutated in long-QT and Jervell-Lange-Nielsen syndromes).

Benign familial infantile convulsions

The syndrome of benign familial infantile convulsions (BFIC) was described as a distinct clinical condition by Vigevano and colleagues in 1992.[10] The onset of seizures occurs usually between four and seven months in infants who are otherwise neurologically and developmentally normal. In the majority, complex partial seizures occur, typically in clusters, over a period of a few days. Seizures remit before the age of 18 months.

The inheritance pattern is autosomal dominant. The mode of inheritance, benign outcome and early age of onset are similar to those of BFNC. These similarities led to the suggestion that BFIC may represent an allelic variant of BFNC. However, linkage studies performed in eight families excluded chromosome 20q as the site of a locus predisposing to BFIC.[11] Linkage analysis performed recently in five Italian pedigrees provided evidence for a locus on chromosome 19q.[12] No evidence for heterogeneity in this family set was obtained.

Partial epilepsy with auditory symptoms

A family in which 11 individuals over three generations had idiopathic partial epilepsy was identified[13] during the ascertainment of patients as part of a large study of the genetic epidemiology of epilepsy. A number of the affected individuals reported auditory disturbance, such as a hum or ringing which grew gradually louder as part of the seizure. The interictal EEG was normal in all cases, and neurological examination was also normal in those who were examined. Linkage analysis was performed in this family, and a locus mapped to chromosome 10q. Further refinement of the localisation of the gene will not be possible without additional families.

Autosomal dominant nocturnal frontal lobe epilepsy

In 1994, five families from Australia, UK and Canada were described with an inherited form of partial epilepsy, autosomal dominant nocturnal frontal lobe epilepsy (ADNFLE).[14] Seizures occurred during sleep and had been misdiagnosed as a variety of conditions including nightmares, night terrors, hysteria, sleep paralysis and paroxysmal nocturnal dystonia. The familial nature of the condition had therefore gone unrecognised. Seizures begin predominantly in childhood and persist into adulthood; they occur in clusters, with brief episodes usually lasting about 60 seconds. The interictal EEG is usually normal, although the ictal EEG may show sharp and slow wave activity in the anterior quadrants bilaterally. Neuroimaging is also normal. The treatment of choice is carbamazepine.

Segregation analysis performed in the five families described supported autosomal dominant inheritance with 69% penetrance and variable expression. Linkage studies performed in a single large Australian pedigree assigned the gene to chromosome 20q13.2, the same region to which *EBN1* maps.[15] However, other families did not appear to be linked to chromosome 20q, indicating the presence of genetic heterogeneity. This region of chromosome 20q contains a candidate gene, *CHRNA4*, which encodes the α4 subunit of the nicotinic acetylcholine receptor. Two different mutations in *CHRNA4* have now been described in two families with ADNFLE:

- a missense mutation that replaces a serine with phenylalanine at codon 248,[16] and
- a three base-pair insertion at position 776.[17]

Both these mutations are thought to result in loss of receptor function. *CHRNA4* was the first gene to be implicated in an idiopathic epilepsy, and led to increased interest in the role of acetylcholine receptor subunits in the brain, as well as rendering this group of genes excellent candidates for involvement in other epilepsy phenotypes.

Non-Mendelian epilepsies

Studies of the genetic basis of the non-Mendelian epilepsies have until recently proved less productive. There is, however, no doubt that these phenotypes will be amenable to genetic analysis given the technological improvements which allow rapid large-scale genome scans. To date, the majority of the studies have concentrated on juvenile myoclonic epilepsy because of its distinctive phenotype and clear genetic predisposition. Few of the other complex epilepsy phenotypes have been subjected to genetic analysis.

Juvenile myoclonic epilepsy

Juvenile myoclonic epilepsy (JME) is a common form of idiopathic generalised epilepsy characterised by myoclonic jerks on awakening. About 90% of affected individuals also have generalised tonic-clonic seizures and 30% have absence seizures. JME is estimated to have a prevalence of between one in 2,000 and one in 4,000. Family studies have demonstrated that 25–30% of the relatives of patients with JME have seizures,[18] a greater proportion than observed for epilepsy as a whole. In a study of 118 patients with JME, Janz *et al*[18] found that 5.5% of first-degree relatives had afebrile seizures (3.4% of parents, 7.1% of siblings and 6.6% of off-spring). About 30% of them also had JME, and the remainder other epilepsy phenotypes.

An estimate of the familial clustering of a disease can be calculated from the ratio of the risk in relatives of patients to the population prevalence (λR).[19] For siblings, the ratio is referred to as λsib or λS. A high value for λR suggests a strong genetic component to disease susceptibility and genetic mapping is relatively straightforward. As the value for λR declines, so does the genetic contribution to the disease and genetic mapping becomes more difficult:

- for epilepsy as a whole: $\lambda S = 0.05/0.005 = 10$;
- for JME: $\lambda S = 0.021/0.0005 = 42$;
- for comparison, λS for type 1 diabetes is 15.

Genetic studies of type 1 diabetes have been successful in identifying a number of susceptibility loci. These figures therefore suggest that it should be possible to identify loci predisposing to JME.

Several studies from two groups have provided evidence for the existence of a locus predisposing to JME and other idiopathic generalised epilepsies on chromosome 6p; the locus has been designated *EJM1*. These studies have, however, failed either to refine the localisation of *EJM1* or to define the epilepsy phenotype to which it predisposes. Liu *et al*[20] have proposed that *EJM1* lies close to the centromere on chromosome 6p and predisposes to 'classical JME' in which absence seizures do not occur. Sander *et al*[21] suggest that *EJM1* confers genetic susceptibility to a broad spectrum of idiopathic generalised epilepsies in families containing an individual with JME and, furthermore, that *EJM1* lies close to the HLA, some distance away from the centromere. Three studies[22–24] have failed to find evidence for the existence of a locus on chromosome 6p. One possible explanation is the presence of genetic heterogeneity, but this has not been formally demonstrated and requires the pooling of resources and data.

Following the identification of mutations in *CHRNA4* in patients with ADNFLE, genes encoding acetylcholine receptor (AChR) subunits became strong candidates for involvement in other epilepsy phenotypes. In a recent study of 34 pedigrees containing two or more relatives with JME, individuals were typed using microsatellite markers encompassing regions of the genome to which AChR subunit genes map. Data were analysed using a new method of combined parametric and non-parametric analysis, GENEHUNTER. The genes which map to chromosomes 1, 8, 15q24 and 20 were excluded, but strong evidence for linkage was obtained in the region on chromosome 15q14 to which *CHRNA7* maps.[25] To date, mutations in *CHRNA7* have not been demonstrated in patients with JME, and it is possible that this region contains other, as yet unidentified, candidate genes.

Idiopathic generalised epilepsy

Zara *et al*[24] investigated 10 families containing 38 affected subjects with a variety of idiopathic generalised epilepsy (IGE) using non-parametric methods of analysis. Regions of the genome previously reported to harbour epilepsy genes were investigated. Using extended sib-pair analysis, the authors found excess of sharing of alleles for three markers on chromosome 8q. The data were also analysed by conventional linkage analysis, and a maximum two-point logarithm of the odds (LOD) score of 1.962 ($\theta = 0.05$)

was obtained at the marker D8S256. The authors suggest that these results provide strongly suggestive evidence for linkage of IGE to chromosome 8q24, but they require replication in an independent data set. The data have been re-analysed by Kruglyak *et al*[26] using GENEHUNTER, with less significant results. There is therefore some doubt over the existence of a locus on chromosome 8q. Zara *et al*[24] note that *EBN2* maps to the same region of chromosome 8q, and speculate that a single locus could predispose to both epilepsy phenotypes. It will be possible to test their hypothesis now that the gene for *EBN2* has been identified.

Febrile convulsions

Although febrile convulsions are not an epileptic syndrome, they are included in the International League Against Epilepsy (ILAE) classification of epilepsies and epileptic syndromes, and susceptibility to them has a strong genetic basis. Estimates of the proportion of probands with an affected relative vary in different studies, with figures between 8% in siblings or parents[27] and 49% in siblings *and* parents being obtained.[28] Linkage analysis was performed in a single large family in which febrile convulsions segregate in an autosomal dominant manner with reduced penetrance.[29] Three subjects also had afebrile seizures. A full genome search was performed and a multipoint LOD score of 3.40 was obtained between the febrile convulsion trait and markers in the region 8q13–21. These results were obtained by maximising the LOD score over a number of models of penetrance and phenocopy rate. They therefore need to be replicated in other families with febrile convulsions.

Conclusion

This chapter has concentrated on those epilepsy phenotypes which have already been the subject of genetic analysis. However, Mendelian epilepsies continue to be described as distinct conditions, and it is certain that the genetic basis of these phenotypes will also be elucidated. Much progress has been made in the analysis of complex phenotypes. Until recently, the complex epilepsies have been a relatively neglected area of genetic research despite epilepsy being a common and distressing disorder with a clear genetic predisposition. The recent identification of genes for the Mendelian epilepsies has sparked a new interest in the complex phenotypes, and it is certain that progress will be made in research into the genetic basis of these conditions.

References

1 Commission on Classification and Terminology of the ILAE. Proposal for revised clinical and electroencephalographic classification of epileptic seizures. *Epilepsia* 1981; **22**: 489–501.

2 Commission on Classification and Terminology of the ILAE. Proposal for revised classification of epilepsies and epilepsy syndromes. *Epilepsia* 1989; **30**: 389–99.

3 Tsuboi T, Christian W. On the genetics of primary generalised epilepsy with sporadic myoclonus of impulsive petit-mal type. *Humangenetik* 1973; **19**: 155–82.

4 Anderson VE, Wilcox KJ, Rich SS, Leppik IE, Hauser WA. Twin studies in epilepsy. In: Beck-Mannagetta G, Anderson VE, Doose H, Janz D (eds). *Genetics of the epilepsies*. Berlin: Springer-Verlag, 1989: 145–55.

5 Leppert M, Anderson VE, Quattlebaum T, Stauffer D, *et al*. Benign familial neonatal convulsions linked to genetic markers on chromosome 20. *Nature* 1989; **337**: 647–8.

6 Ryan SG, Wiznitzer M, Hollman C, Torres M, *et al*. Benign familial neonatal convulsions: evidence for clinical and genetic heterogeneity. *Annals of Neurology* 1991; **29**: 469–73.

7 Lewis TB, Leach RJ, Ward K, O'Connell P, Ryan SG. Genetic heterogeneity in benign familial neonatal convulsions: identification of a new locus on chromosome 8q. *American Journal of Human Genetics* 1993; **53**: 670–5.

8 Singh NA, Charlier C, Stauffer D, Dupont BR, *et al*. A novel potassium channel gene, KCNQ2, is mutated in an inherited epilepsy of newborns. *Nature Genetics* 1998; **18**: 25–9.

9 Charlier C, Singh NA, Ryan SG, Lewis TB, *et al*. A pore mutation in a novel KQT-like potassium channel gene in an idiopathic epilepsy family. *Nature Genetics* 1998; **18**: 53–5.

10 Vigevano F, Fusco L, Di Capua M, Ricci S, *et al*. Benign infantile familial convulsions. *European Journal of Paediatrics* 1992; **151**: 608–12.

11 Malafosse A, Beck C, Bellet H, DiCapua M, *et al*. Benign infantile familial convulsions are not an allelic form of the benign familial neonatal convulsions gene. *Annals of Neurology* 1994; **35**: 479–82.

12 Guipponi M, Rivier F, Vigevano F, Beck C, *et al*. Linkage mapping of benign infantile convulsions (BFIC) to chromosome 19q. *Human Molecular Genetics* 1997; **6**: 473–7.

13 Ottman R, Risch N, Hauser WA, Pedley TA, *et al*. Localization of a gene for partial epilepsy to chromosome 10q. *Nature Genetics* 1995; **10**: 56–60.

14 Scheffer IE, Bhatia KP, Lopes-Cendes I, Fish DR, *et al*. Autosomal dominant frontal epilepsy misdiagnosed as sleep disorder. *Lancet* 1994; **343**: 515–7.

15 Phillips HA, Scheffer IE, Berkovic SF, Hollway GE, *et al*. Localization of a gene for autosomal dominant nocturnal frontal lobe epilepsy to chromosome 20q13.2. *Nature Genetics* 1995; **10**: 117–8.

16 Steinlein OK, Mulley JC, Propping P, Wallace RH, *et al*. A missense mutation in the neuronal receptor a4 subunit is associated with autosomal dominant nocturnal frontal lobe epilepsy. *Nature Genetics* 1995; **11**: 201–3.

17 Steinlein OK, Magnusson A, Stoodt J, Bertrand S, *et al.* An insertion mutation of the CHRNA4 gene in a family with autosomal dominant nocturnal frontal lobe epilepsy. *Human Molecular Genetics* 1997; **6**: 943–7.

18 Janz D, Durner M, Beck-Mannagetta G, Pantazis G. Family studies on the genetics of juvenile myoclonic epilepsy (epilepsy with impulsive petit mal). In: Beck-Mannagetta G, Anderson VE, Doose H, Janz D (eds). *Genetics of the epilepsies.* Berlin: Springer-Verlag, 1989: 43–52.

19 Risch N. Linkage strategies for genetically complex traits. I. Multilocus models. *American Journal of Human Genetics* 1990; **46**: 222–8.

20 Liu AW, Delgado-Escueta AV, Serratosa JM, Alonso ME, *et al.* Juvenile myoclonic epilepsy locus in chromosome 6p21.2–p11: linkage to convulsions and electroencephalography trait. *American Journal of Human Genetics* 1995; **57**: 368–81.

21 Sander T, Hildmann BC, Janz D, Wienker TF, *et al.* The phenotypic spectrum related to the human epilepsy susceptibility gene 'EJM1'. *Annals of Neurology* 1995; **38**: 210–7.

22 Whitehouse WP, Rees M, Curtis D, Sundqvist A, *et al.* Linkage analysis of idiopathic generalised epilepsy (IGE) and marker loci on chromosome 6p in families of patients with juvenile myoclonic epilepsy: no evidence for an epilepsy locus in the HLA region. *American Journal of Human Genetics* 1993; **53**: 652–62.

23 Elmslie FV, Williamson MP, Rees M, Kerr M, *et al.* Linkage analysis of juvenile myoclonic epilepsy and microsatellite loci spanning 61 cM of human chromosome 6p in 19 nuclear pedigrees provides no evidence for a susceptibility locus in this region. *American Journal of Human Genetics* 1996; **59**: 653–63.

24 Zara F, Bianchi A, Avanzini G, Di Donato S, *et al.* Mapping of genes predisposing to idiopathic generalized epilepsy. *Human Molecular Genetics* 1995; **4**: 1201–7.

25 Elmslie FV, Rees M, Williamson MP, Kerr M, *et al.* Genetic mapping of a major susceptibility locus for juvenile myoclonic epilepsy on chromosome 15q. *Human Molecular Genetics* 1997; **6**: 1329–34.

26 Kruglyak L, Daly MJ, Reeve-Daly MP, Lander ES. Parametric and non-parametric linkage analysis: a unified multipoint approach. *American Journal of Human Genetics* 1996; **58**: 1347–63.

27 Rich SS, Annegers JF, Hauser WA, Anderson VE. Complex segregation analysis of febrile convulsions. *American Journal of Human Genetics* 1987; **41**: 249–57.

28 Wallace SJ. Genetic factors. In: Wallace SJ (ed). *The child with febrile seizures.* London: John Wright, 1988: 24–31.

29 Wallace RH, Berkovic SF, Howell RA, Sutherland GR, Mulley JC. Suggestion of a major gene for familial febrile convulsions mapping to 8q13–21. *Journal of Medical Genetics* 1996; **33**: 308–12.

16 | Predisposing genes, high-risk environments and coronary artery disease: lipoprotein lipase and fibrinogen as examples

Steve Humphries, Rachel Fisher, Philippa Talmud
Cardiovascular Genetics, Department of Medicine,
University College London Medical School

George Miller
Wolfson Institute, St Bartholomew's Hospital, London

Hugh Montgomery
Hatter Institute for Cardiovascular Studies,
University College London Medical School

Coronary artery disease (CAD) is a multifactorial disorder, with both genetic and environmental factors involved to varying extents. Epidemiological studies have identified a number of these factors, including high blood pressure, smoking, high dietary fat intake, obesity and the development of diabetes. These studies have also identified a number of plasma risk factors such as elevated levels of cholesterol, triglyceride (TG)[1] and the clotting factor fibrinogen.[2] Information at the level of genotype may provide additional understanding:

- When a genotype predicts a level of a measurable risk factor at some future time, such as the change in plasma lipid levels with the development of obesity or diabetes, increasing age or following infection or injury;
- Where the gene codes for a protein are not easily measurable, for example, in heart muscle, the intestine, the liver or cells in the vessel wall.

Examples of the first type of genotype information will be presented in this chapter.

The critical role of genes is in coding for the structural proteins and enzymes which enable the cell, organ or organism to maintain homoeostasis in the face of the environmental challenges experienced. Genetic variation within a population will mean that individuals have different ability to maintain homoeostasis when faced with a specific environmental challenge. The clinical features of any disorder with a late age of onset can therefore be thought of as being caused by the failure of the individual to maintain homoeostasis. This is particularly true for the disorder of CAD. Thus, for any individual in the general population, the level of a risk factor in the blood such as TG or fibrinogen is due to that individual's genetically determined ability to maintain homoeostasis in response to the environment being experienced. The current epidemic of CAD being seen in Western societies is mainly due to an inability in some individuals to maintain optimum blood levels of these risk-factor components, in the light of the environment experienced as a result of 'affluent' lifestyle changes, such as dietary fat intake, the development of obesity or cigarette smoking.

Plasma triglycerides, lipoprotein lipase variants and obesity

A growing body of evidence supports the hypothesis that elevated plasma TG levels may increase the risk of CAD. Lipoprotein lipase (LPL) is a key enzyme in the metabolism of TG-rich lipoproteins by hydrolysing TGs in large TG-rich lipoproteins (chylomicrons and very low density lipoproteins). To date, two common missense mutations have been identified in the *LPL* gene (for review see Ref 3):

- Aspartic acid to asparagine change in exon 2 (D9N). *In vitro*, LPL-N9 demonstrates a 20–30% decrease in mass with retention in the cells, suggesting a secretion defect.[4]
- Asparagine to serine change (N291S) in exon 6. *In vitro*, LPL-S291 demonstrates reduced dimer stability, with overall 30–50% reduced activity.

We examined the effect of the mutations on plasma lipid levels in 628 healthy individuals who were participating in the Northwick Park Heart Study II, a prospective study of healthy men in the UK.[5] In this group, 27 LPL-N9 and 24 LPL-S291 carriers were identified,[6,7] with plasma TG levels 24% and 14% higher, respectively, than individuals with neither mutation. The relationship of body-mass index (BMI) (divided according to tertiles) with plasma TG concentration in carriers and non-carriers is shown in Fig 1. In the non-carriers, there was the expected graded increase in plasma

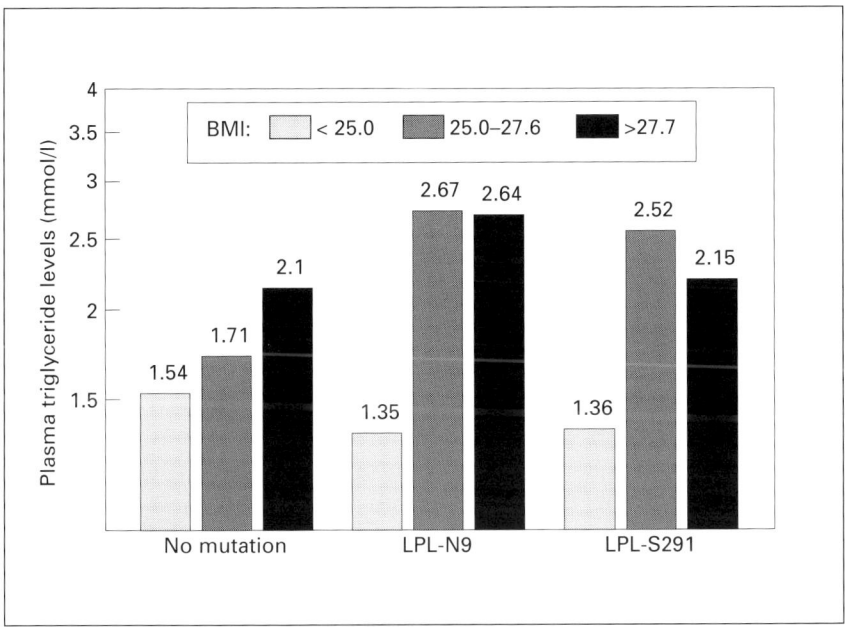

Fig 1. *Mean plasma triglyceride concentration according to tertiles of body-mass index (BMI) in healthy non-carriers and carriers of the LPL-N9 (n=26) or LPL-S291 (n=24) lipoprotein lipase (LPL) mutation.* For carriers of either mutation, the test for interaction between carriers/non-carriers and tertiles of BMI was $p = 0.006$. To test differences in triglyceride levels, values were log-transformed prior to statistical analysis (from Refs 6 and 7).

TG across the BMI tertiles. In carriers of either mutation, there was a much greater increase in plasma TG concentration in the upper two BMI tertile groups compared to the lowest BMI tertile group. Thus, both variants are implicated in causing elevated plasma TG concentrations which are exaggerated at higher BMI. Obesity may promote overproduction of TG-rich lipoproteins from the liver, which overwhelms the partially deficient LPL in the adipose and muscle. Carriers of these LPL mutations who are also moderately obese would therefore be at increased risk of CAD. An association between greater risk of CAD events and being a carrier of either LPL-N9[8] or LPL-S291[9] has recently been reported.

Variability at the fibrinogen locus and plasma fibrinogen levels

The three fibrinogen genes are in a cluster of less than 50 kb on the long arm of chromosome 4, and each chain is synthesised as a separate messenger RNA (mRNA), with the levels of all three mRNAs coordinately controlled. The rate-limiting step in the production of the mature fibrinogen molecule in the human hepatoma cell-line HepG2 is the synthesis of the Bβ-polypeptide chain,[10] which in turn is influenced by the amount of its mRNA available. It is therefore likely that an alteration in the level of the Bβ-chain synthesis may have an effect on the amount of fibrinogen secreted by the liver.

β-gene promoter

The structure of the β-gene promoter has been well studied. The region from −150 bp to the start of transcription appears to contain all the information required to act as a promoter in HepG2 cells, and has been shown to bind proteins from a HepG2 cell nuclear extract. The sequence from −89 to −76 contains a conserved liver-specific transcription element which binds hepatic nuclear factor 1 (HNF1). Deletion mapping shows that just upstream lies an interleukin (IL) 6 responsive element (IL6RE),[11] which has been identified in other genes as the motif CTGGGA. It is therefore possible that sequence changes in this region of the gene may have a direct effect on the rate of transcription and thus on plasma fibrinogen levels.

In studies of the β-fibrinogen promoter,[12] we detected a common G/A sequence variation at position −455, with the A present in approximately 20% of alleles examined. In more than 10 independent studies from five different laboratories with samples of more than 20,000 healthy individuals the A^{-455} allele has been consistently associated with higher fibrinogen levels.[13–15] Those with one or more copies of the A^{-455} allele have, on average, 0.28 g/l higher fibrinogen levels than those with the genotype G/G (weighted average in healthy men, see Ref 15).

The magnitude of this genotype effect indicates that it is likely to be of biological significance in causing an elevated risk of thrombosis. By extrapolation from the prospective data[2] of the relationship between fibrinogen and ischaemic heart disease risk (0.6 g/l associated with 84% greater risk), men with the A allele would be at 40% higher risk of a thrombotic event. This estimate is based on healthy middle-aged men from north London, and may not be the same in other groups.

Although the A^{-455} sequence is outside the region of the reported promoter sequence, it is possible that it has a direct effect on transcription, and preliminary studies have demonstrated binding of a hepatic nuclear protein to the G but not to the A sequence.[16] However, it has recently been found that the $G^{-455} \rightarrow A$ sequence change in all Caucasian populations studied to date is in complete allelic association with a $C^{-148} \rightarrow T$ change located close to the consensus sequence of the IL6 element.[17] This raises the possibility that the $G \rightarrow A$ change acts as a neutral marker for the $C \rightarrow T$ change, which is the functional change working through effects on transcription of the β-fibrinogen gene mediated by IL6: that is, the T^{-148} sequence close to the IL6RE may increase the affinity of NF-IL6, leading to enhanced transcription of the β-fibrinogen gene. Experiments are in progress to insert this fragment of the gene into the appropriate vector to test this hypothesis.

Acute phase stimulation of fibrinogen by exercise

Fibrinogen is an acute phase protein and its plasma level is raised following infection or injury. Because of its sensitivity to environmental factors, there is a high within-individual variation of fibrinogen levels. It is possible that some individuals in the general population may have a 'plastic' genotype that responds easily to environmental factors, and would experience a greater than average increase in plasma fibrinogen levels in response to a moderate environmental stimulus. They would then be at greater than average risk of a thrombotic event at the peak of fibrinogen levels, and thus have a greater chance of developing CAD, particularly myocardial infarction (MI).

To investigate this further, we examined the effects of acute intensive exercise on plasma fibrinogen levels and the relationship of these responses to genotype in 156 male British Army recruits.[18] They were studied at the start of their 10-week basic training (which emphasises physical fitness) and at 0.5–5 days after a major two-day strenuous military exercise (ME). At day 5 after the ME, fibrinogen concentrations were significantly lower than at baseline (12%, $p = 0.04$), consistent with the beneficial effect of training. However, within 12 hours of the completion of the exercise, fibrinogen levels were 14.5% higher than at five days, suggesting that the acute response had already begun. Levels were significantly higher on days 1–3 after ME (suggesting an 'acute phase' response to strenuous exercise) and maximal on days 1 and 2 (27% and 37%, respectively, $p < 0.001$). The duration of the rise (at least 3 days) may be related to either continued fibrinogen production or its long plasma half-life (4.5–6.5 days), but the time course of this response was similar to that seen after the physiological stress of MI.[19]

The fibrinogen-raising effect associated with the A allele was seen at baseline and after five days, but the effect was modest and non-significant in this small sample. In particular, it can be noted

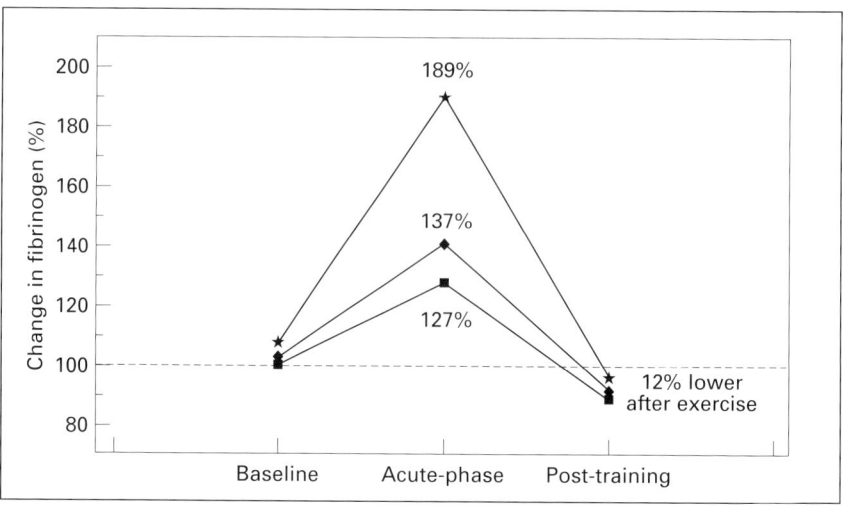

Fig 2. *Mean percentage change in plasma fibrinogen in young men before (pre-training) and after severe exercise (2–3 days and five days following an intensive two-day military exercise) by fibrinogen G/A genotype (—■— = GG; —□— = GA; —✻— = AA) (from Ref 17).*

that the ranking of the three genotypes was similar before and after training, raising the possibility that the beneficial effects of training in lowering fibrinogen levels may be due to increases in fibrinolysis (and therefore not related to fibrinogen genotype) rather than to reduced synthesis. However, as shown in Fig 2, the degree of rise at 2–3 days after ME was strongly related to the presence of the A allele. Although the group was small, the differences were statistically significant ($p = 0.01$), and the size of the effect sufficient to be of biological significance. In particular, the men homozygous for the A allele (representing 4% of the population based on the observed allele frequencies) had fibrinogen levels which by day 2 had risen by more than 100% compared to their 'untrained' levels, and were amongst the highest levels in the whole sample. These findings support an association of the A allele with greater fibrinogen level 'responsiveness' after a cytokine inducing event.

Conclusions

We have described two genetic predictors for an individual's CAD risk, which may be useful over and above that of measures of classical risk factors. For the LPL variants, the modest reduction of lipolytic action appears likely to be important particularly when individuals are also overweight. The clinical implication for obese carriers of these variants is that they may experience a large and clinically useful reduction in TG concentration for a moderate loss of weight. For the fibrinogen gene, the molecular mechanisms underlying the associations and environmental interactions are likely to be due to changes in the transcription of the β-fibrinogen gene in response to cytokine-mediated stimuli such as smoking, inflammation and tissue damage. The magnitude of the response raises the possibility that individuals homozygous for the fibrinogen A allele may be at particular risk of a thrombotic event following, for example, an acute phase stimulus, or the development of diabetes. Once identified, such individuals may benefit from risk factor reduction. Further work is required to explore whether similar gene/environment interaction occurs in individuals of different ethnic origin, in both men and women, and in those with different forms of vascular disease. When the mechanisms controlling changes in plasma risk factors in response to personal environmental changes are better understood, it may also be possible to develop directed therapeutic strategies that will reduce risk in a genotype-specific manner, for example where levels of fibrinogen gene transcription may be modulated by specific antagonists of nuclear protein binding.

Acknowledgements

This work was supported by the British Heart Foundation (PG007 and 86–77) and by the Medical Research Council (GJM).

References

1   Bainton D, Miller NE, Bolton CH, Yarnell JW, *et al*. Plasma triglyceride and high density lipoprotein cholesterol as predictors of ischaemic heart disease in British men: the Caerphilly and Speedwell Collaborative Heart Disease Studies. *British Heart Journal* 1992; **68**: 60–6.

2   Meade TW, Mellows S, Brozovic M, Miller GJ, *et al*. Haemostatic function and ischaemic heart disease: principal results of the Northwick Park Heart Study. *Lancet* 1986; **ii**: 533–7.

3   Fisher RM, Humphries SE, Talmud PJ. Common variation in the lipoprotein lipase gene: effects on plasma lipids and risk of atherosclerosis. *Atherosclerosis* 1997; **135**: 145–59.

4   Zhang H, Henderson H, Gagne SE, Clee SM, *et al*. Common sequence variants of lipoprotein lipase: standardized studies of in vitro expression and catalytic function. *Biochimica et Biophysica Acta* 1996; **1302**: 159–66.

5 Miller GJ, Bauer KA, Barzegar S, Cooper JA, Rosenberg RD. Increased activation of the haemostatic system in men at high risk of fatal coronary heart disease. *Thrombosis and Haemostasis* 1996; **75**: 767–71.

6 Mailly F, Tugrul Y, Reymer PWA, Bruin T, *et al*. A common variant in the gene for lipoprotein lipase (Asp9→Asn): functional implications and prevalence in normal and hyperlipidemic subjects. *Arteriosclerosis, Thrombosis and Vascular Biology* 1995; **15**: 468–78.

7 Fisher RM, Mailly F, Peacock RE, Hamsten A, *et al*. Interaction of the lipoprotein lipase asparagine 291→serine mutation with body mass index determines elevated plasma triacylglycerol concentrations: a study in hyperlipidaemic subjects, myocardial infarction survivors and healthy adults. *Journal of Lipid Research* 1995; **36**: 2104–12.

8 Jukema JW, van Boven AJ, Groenemeijer B, Zwinderman AH, *et al*. The Asp9→Asn mutation in the lipoprotein lipase gene is associated with increased progression of coronary atherosclerosis. *Circulation* 1996; **94**: 1913.

9 Wittrup HW, Tybjaerg-Hansen A, Abildgaard S, Steffensen R, *et al*. A common substitution (Asn291Ser) in lipoprotein lipase is associated with increased risk of ischaemic heart disease. *Journal of Clinical Investigation* 1997; **99**: 1606.

10 Roy SN, Mukhopadhyay G, Redman CM. Regulation of fibrinogen assembly. Transfection of HepG2 cells with Bβ cDNA specifically enhances synthesis of the three component chains of fibrinogen. *Journal of Biological Chemistry* 1990; **265**: 6389–93.

11 Dalmon J, Laurent M, Courtois G. The human β fibrinogen promoter contains a hepatocyte nuclear factor 1-dependent interleukin-6 responsive element. *Molecular and Cellular Biology* 1993; **13**: 1183–93.

12 Thomas A, Kelleher C, Green F, Meade TW, Humphries SE. Variation in the promoter region of the β-fibrinogen gene is associated with plasma fibrinogen levels in smokers and non-smokers. *Thrombosis and Haemostasis* 1991; **65**: 487–90.

13 Humphries S, Ye S, Talmud P, Bara L, *et al*. European Atherosclerosis Research Study. Genotype at the fibrinogen locus (G_{-455}-A β-gene) is associated with differences in plasma fibrinogen levels in young men and women from different regions in Europe: evidence for gender-genotype-environment interaction. *Arteriosclerosis, Thrombosis and Vascular Biology* 1995; **15**: 96-104.

14 Tybjaerg-Hansen A, Agerholm-Larsen B, Humphries SE, Abildgaard S, *et al*. A common mutation (G-455→A) in the β-*fibrinogen* promoter is an independent predictor of plasma fibrinogen, but not of ischemic heart disease. A study of 9,127 individuals based on the Copenhagen City Heart Study. *Journal of Clinical Investigation* 1997; **99**: 3034–9.

15 Humphries SE, Green F, Thomas A, Montgomery HE, *et al*. Gene-environment interaction in the determination of plasma fibrinogen levels. *Fibrinolysis and Proteolysis* 1997; **11**(Suppl 1): 3–7.

16 Lane A, Humphries SE, Green FR. Effect on transcription of two common genetic polymorphisms adjacent to the promoter region of the B-fibrinogen gene. *Thrombosis and Haemostasis* 1993; **69**: 1539.

17   Thomas A, Lamlum H, Humphries S, Green F. Linkage disequilibrium across the fibrinogen locus as shown by five genetic polymorphisms, G/A^{-455} (HaeIII), C/T^{-148} (HindIII/AluI), T/G^{-1689} (AvaII), and BclI (β-fibrinogen) and TaqI (α-fibrinogen), and their detection by PCR. *Human Mutation* 1994; **3**: 79–81.

18   Montgomery HE, Clarkson P, Nwose OM, Mikalidis DP, *et al*. The acute rise in serum fibrinogen concentration with exercise is influenced by the G-453-A polymorphism of the beta-fibrinogen gene. *Arteriosclerosis, Thrombosis and Vascular Biology* 1996; **16**: 386–91.

19   Haines AP, Howarth D, North WRS, Goldenberg E, *et al*. Haemostatic variables and outcome of acute myocardial infarction. *Thrombosis and Haemostasis* 1983; **50**: 800–3.

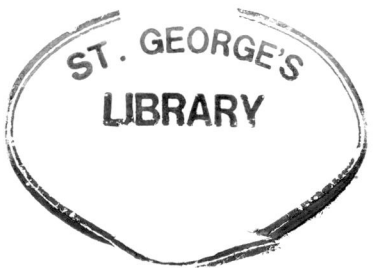

Part 5

Future prospects

17 | Developmental biology

Veronica van Heyningen
Cell Genetics Section, MRC Human Genetics Unit,
Western General Hospital, Edinburgh, and Faculty of Medicine,
University of Edinburgh

Developmental anomalies are very common in all human populations. A high proportion arise as a result of inherited or *de novo* mutations, but some are caused by teratogenic environmental effects. A few are simply the result of stochastic processes going wrong in the course of that most complex of processes, the development of the multicellular organism from a single fertilised cell. Development needs to be both precise and highly plastic, so what is amazing is not that it sometimes goes wrong but that it is *ever* successful.

The interactions of many genes are involved in each step in the progression, and they are difficult to unravel – although sophisticated transplantation and ablation experiments have made major contributions to our current level of knowledge. In recent years, the observations derived from the study of mutations have been most illuminating in revealing how normal development should proceed through showing how it goes wrong when a particular cog in the machine is not working properly.

A closely observed and documented human population is the best source of mutations for the study of the range of developmental anomalies. No other model system with the largest and most minute of mutation screens will provide a better resource but, to understand the components of the developmental machinery, it is usually necessary to move to model organisms for experimental analysis. Until recently, all but a few visionaries felt that to unravel developmental pathways it was necessary to use a mammalian system as close as possible to man. However, the tremendous conservation of genes and pathways throughout evolution has now become clear, so we can now contemplate using many different organisms to dissect gene interactions and generally understand gene function.

A great deal can be learnt about which key genes are involved in which process by studying human malformations and inherited developmental variations. Clinicians can contribute enormously to this process by observing patients closely, taking accurate and detailed family histories, and describing phenotypes minutely. It is also important to document cases in an accessible way and, where there is some prospect of imminent genetic analysis, useful to collect some tissue samples, usually peripheral lymphocytes, which can be used to make DNA and stored for permanent cell-line transformation with Epstein-Barr virus.

Genes implicated in developmental abnormalities

It may be easier to find the genes implicated in developmental abnormalities by asking what kinds of genes are *not* so involved. Many different classes of genes have been shown to be mutated in different developmental diseases, but some types turn up more often than others (Table 1). When researchers are thinking about possible candidate genes for specific diseases, they frequently think most readily about transcriptional regulators – DNA-binding proteins known to be involved in regulating the expression of a number of downstream genes, and hence in regulating whole pathways.

Genetics of developmental abnormalities

All types of inheritance patterns can be associated with developmental anomalies: autosomal dominant, autosomal recessive, sex-linked (X and Y). Quite a high proportion of cases are sporadic, due to new mutations, in some cases of such severe effect that the affected individuals never reproduce.

Table 1. Classes of genes frequently associated with developmental anomalies.

- DNA-binding transcription factors
- RNA-binding proteins with a role in RNA processing
- Receptors: cell surface, intracellular, nuclear
- Ligands: growth factors, hormones
- Channels, transporters, cell junction proteins
- Extracellular matrix molecules
- Chromatin regulators
- DNA repair enzymes

Haploinsufficiency diseases

One interesting category, seen perhaps more often in humans than might be expected from other well-studied genetic organisms like Drosophila (and even perhaps the mouse), is the so-called 'haploinsufficiency' diseases. These present as apparently dominant mutations, but result specifically from a complete functional loss of one copy of the gene. It must be deduced that the developing organism is highly sensitive to a 50% loss of active gene product in these cases. It is not unusual to observe more than one disease phenotype resulting from mutations with different effects at a single locus. An excellent recent example is provided by the *GLI3* gene with distinct classes of mutation giving rise to Greig cephalopolysyndactyly, Pallister-Hall syndrome and postaxial polydactyly type A.[1]

Identifying new disease genes by chromosomal position

There are many different approaches to identifying appropriate candidate genes. Perhaps one of the most successful has been the positional candidate approach (a hybrid of the 'positional cloning' and 'candidate gene' approaches described in Chapter 13), in which the approximate position of the gene has been identified by family linkage studies or through the observation of chromosomal rearrangements (deletions, translocations, inversions). The chromosomal region is then studied in detail to search for genes within it. Any genes already assigned to the region that appear to be possible disease loci on the basis of predicted function and expression pattern are then looked at in detail for mutations in affected cases. This can be laborious, but has led to the identification of a good number of diseases genes. Examples include:

- The identification of the inhibitory glycine receptor alpha subunit as gene-mutated in startle disease;[2]
- *PAX3* in Waardenburg syndrome type I,[3] although here there was the additional help of suggested homology between the mouse *Splotch* mutation and this human pigmentary disturbance,[4] and the fact that the *Pax3* gene had just been shown to be mutated in these mice.
- Waardenburg syndrome type II was similarly shown by Read's group to result from mutation at the *MITF* locus,[5] which is also involved in mouse microphthalmia.

PAX3 and *MITF* represent two different classes of transcription factors with a role in neural crest cell migration, which is faulty in both types of Waardenburg syndrome and in the mouse anomalies. Waardenburg syndrome is a good example of genetic heterogeneity where very similar phenotypes are caused by mutations at different loci.

This positional approach still involves much hard work in most cases because there is not yet a comprehensive gene map for all regions of the genome. As human genome sequencing progresses, the pinpointing of candidate genes should become much easier.

Analysis of genomic regions

There are a number of cases where only arduous analysis of large genomic regions revealed the gene responsible for interesting developmental anomalies. The identification of the chromosome 11p13-linked aniridia gene *PAX6*,[6] another paired box containing transcription factor, and the nearby zinc finger gene, the Wilms' tumour predisposition gene *WT1*,[7] both fall into this category. More recently, a nuclear protein *EYA1*, which may well be a transcription factor, was identified at 8q13.3 as the gene responsible for branchio-oto-renal syndrome.[8] The male sex determination gene, *SRY*, required for testis determination, was one of the prime examples of a gene isolated purely on the basis of chromosomal localisation (reviewed in Ref 9).

In each of these cases the expression pattern had to be compatible with the disease phenotype. However, some of these same examples illustrate clearly that the expression pattern does not always coincide fully with the pattern of disease-associated abnormalities, which often affect only a subset of the expressing tissues.

Expression pattern suggests candidate disease

Sometimes knowledge of expression pattern alone can suggest candidate disease(s) in which to look for mutations at that locus. One impressive example of this is the finding of heterozygous point mutations in cases of schizencephaly in the *EMX2* gene, a highly anteriorly expressed homeobox gene.[10] Another good illustration of how well this approach can work is the association of *PAX2* mutations in renal coloboma syndrome with familial optic nerve colobomas, renal hypoplasia, vesicoureteral reflux, and occasional sensorineural deafness.[11]

Mouse knock-outs provide clues

Sometimes there is no naturally occurring mouse model to provide phenotypic clues and a more amenable genetic system for homing in on the gene by mapping. New, often severe, mouse phenotypes are increasingly being created by so-called gene knock-outs. The interest of the gene is quite frequently suggested by awareness of a similar Drosophila gene.

HOX genes

One of the first series of genes to be studied intensively by creating loss-of-function mutations were the homologues of the original set of Drosophila homoeotic genes, now named *HOX* genes in humans, which are implicated in defining the antero-posterior body axis and its differentiation. In many cases, little or no mouse abnormality was seen, even when both copies were knocked out. Some *Hox* gene knock-outs revealed much more severe effects when crossed with mice carrying homozygous loss at a second *Hox* locus.[12] Recently, however, heterozygous *Hoxa13* loss of function has been implicated in mouse and human malformations in hypo-dactyly[13] and in human hand-foot-genital syndrome.[14]

Hedgehog genes

Other genes of critical interest are the major diffusible signalling genes of Drosophila, hedgehog (*hh*), wingless and their receptors. Mammals have four or more *hedgehog* genes, the best known being *sonic hedgehog* (*SHH*) which is involved in central nervous system development. The homozygotes for *Shh* knock-out in mice are highly abnormal and die *in utero*, with phenotypes resembling severe holoprosencephaly (HPE) in humans.[15] *HPE3* was mapped to a region of chromosome 7 which is also the site for *SHH*. After some initial concerns about a few HPE-associated translocation cases which lay close to, but did not disrupt, the *SHH* gene,[16] mutations in *SHH* were demonstrated in several HPE cases.[17] In such situations, the chromosomal rearrangement is thought to prevent gene expression at a distance by disturbing correct chromosomal organisation (briefly referred to as position effects). As with all other types of mutations, the aberrant disease-associated gene expression can provide much insight into normal control of gene function.

The accumulating mouse gene knock-out phenotypes should continue to help in understanding some mysterious, cruel and all too frequent diseases such as neural tube defects; for example, it remains to be seen whether the variable, but unmistakable failure to close the neural tube properly in the mouse knock-outs for the *Cart1* homoeobox gene has any bearing on some of the similar human abnormalities.[18] However, the mouse phenotype can be modulated by folic acid treatment, which could provide some understanding of the nutritional conditions that need to be established to prevent at least some neural tube defects.

Model organisms: man is the richest resource

The mouse is not the only animal model amenable to complex manipulation, allowing the creation of developmental abnormalities that mirror human disease. As the genome programme continues, it becomes increasingly obvious that many developmental pathways and the genes involved in the necessary interactions have been highly conserved throughout evolution, from yeast and fruitflies to man. Thus, the most experimentally appropriate organism can often be chosen to explore how genes work, how their mutations cause developmental disease and, perhaps increasingly, to work out rational therapeutic approaches to the management of analogous conditions in man.[19] It is, however, unlikely that all human disease phenotypes will be readily recreated in other organisms. The well observed, well preserved human population is ultimately the best source of the broadest spectrum of developmental anomalies capable of providing insight into the aetiology of human disease and its management. Correlation of clinically well observed phenotype with molecularly defined mutational genotype can provide significant biological insight into disease mechanisms. It can also give important information on prognosis in progressive conditions, such as degenerative disease and cancer predisposition.[20] To improve understanding and management of developmental abnormalities, it is essential to foster strong collaborations between clinicians and molecular and functional biologists.

References

1 Biesecker LG. Strike three for GLI3. *Nature Genetics* 1997; **17**: 259–60.
2 Shiang R, Ryan SG, Zhu YZ, Hahn AF, *et al.* Mutations in the alpha 1 subunit of the inhibitory glycine receptor cause the dominant neurologic disorder, hyperekplexia. *Nature Genetics* 1993; **5**: 351–8.
3 Tassabehji M, Read AP, Newton VE, Harris R, *et al.* Waardenburg's syndrome patients have mutations in the human homologue of the Pax-3 paired box gene. *Nature* 1992; **355**: 635–6.
4 Foy C, Newton V, Wellesley D, Harris R, Read AP. Assignment of the locus for Waardenburg syndrome type I to human chromosome 2q37

and possible homology to the Splotch mouse. *American Journal of Human Genetics* 1990; **46**: 1017–23.

5   Tassabehji M, Newton VE, Read AP. Waardenburg syndrome type 2 caused by mutations in the human microphthalmia (MITF) gene. *Nature Genetics* 1994; **8**: 251–5.

6   Ton CCT, Hirvonen H, Miwa H, Weil MM, *et al.* Positional cloning and characterization of a paired box- and homeobox-containing gene from the aniridia region. *Cell* 1991; **67**: 1059–74.

7   Call KM, Glaser T, Ito CY, Buckler AJ, *et al.* Isolation and characterization of a zinc finger polypeptide gene at the human chromosome 11 Wilms' tumour locus. *Cell* 1990; **60**: 509–20.

8   Abdelhak S, Kalatzis V, Heilig R, Compain S, *et al.* A human homologue of the Drosophila eyes absent gene underlies branchio-oto-renal (BOR) syndrome and identifies novel gene family. *Nature Genetics* 1997; **15**: 157–64.

9   Goodfellow PN, Lovell-Badge R. SRY and sex determination in mammals. *Annual Review of Genetics* 1993; **27**: 71–92.

10   Brunelli S, Faiella A, Capra V, Nigro V, *et al.* Germline mutations in the homeobox gene EMX2 in patients with severe schizencephaly. *Nature Genetics* 1996; **12**: 94–6.

11   Sanyanusin P, Schimmenti LA, McNoe LA, Ward TA, *et al.* Mutation of the PAX2 gene in a family with optic nerve colobomas, renal anomalies and vesicoureteral reflux. *Nature Genetics* 1995; **9**: 358–63.

12   Davis AP, Witte DP, Hsieh-Li HM, Potter SS, Capecchi MR. Absence of radius and ulna in mice lacking hoxa-11 and hoxd-11. *Nature* 1995; **375**: 791–5.

13   Mortlock DP, Post LC, Innis JW. The molecular basis of hypodactyly (Hd): a deletion in Hoxa 13 leads to arrest of digital arch formation. *Nature Genetics* 1996; **13**: 284–9.

14   Mortlock DP, Innis JW. Mutation of HOXA13 in hand-foot-genital syndrome. *Nature Genetics* 1997; **15**: 179–80.

15   Chiang C, Litingtung Y, Lee E, Young KE, *et al.* Cyclopia and defective axial patterning in mice lacking sonic hedgehog gene function. *Nature* 1996; **383**: 407–13.

16   Belloni E, Muenke M, Roessler E, Traverso G, *et al.* Identification of sonic hedgehog as a candidate gene responsible for holoprosencephaly. *Nature Genetics* 1996; **14**: 353–6.

17   Roessler E, Belloni E, Gaudenz K, Jay P, *et al.* Mutations in the human sonic hedgehog gene cause holoprosencephaly. *Nature Genetics* 1996; **14**: 357–60.

18   Zhao Q, Behringer RR, de Crombrugghe B. Prenatal folic acid treatment suppresses acrania and meroanencephaly in mice mutant for the Cart1 homeobox gene. *Nature Genetics* 1996; **13**: 275–83.

19   van Heyningen V. Model organisms illuminate human genetics and disease. *Molecular Medicine* 1997; **3**: 231–7.

20   van Heyningen V. Sugar and spice and all things splice? *Nature Genetics* 1997; **17**: 367–8.

18 | Gene therapy

David Porteous
Molecular Genetics Section, MRC Human Genetics Unit,
Western General Hospital, Edinburgh

The promise of gene discovery

From piecemeal beginnings in the 1980s, the Human Genome Project has rapidly shaped into the biggest science project of the 1990s. Gene discovery will lead to a better understanding of the biology underlying health and disease. Beyond the immediate benefits in terms of better diagnosis and preventive treatment, there is the firm expectation that new treatments will emerge, including correction of basic defects by gene therapy.[1] For many individuals and families affected by rare inherited disorders, a cure by gene therapy is the 'Holy Grail'. Gene therapy has also caught the media's attention and the public's imagination. However, reports of a 'breakthrough' are often soon followed by suggestions that 'gene therapy isn't working'. In truth, reality currently lies somewhere in between.

Scientific and practical problems facing gene therapy

The attraction of gene therapy is the simplicity of the concept, as illustrated by severe combined immune deficiency due to a single gene defect resulting in a lack of the enzyme adenosine deaminase (ADA) (reviewed in Refs 2 and 3). The gene is cloned and small enough to be packaged into a retrovirus. Retroviruses can infect bone marrow stem cells, the infected cells can divide, differentiate and enter the circulation. It follows that if the ADA gene is switched on, the immune deficiency will be corrected. ADA deficiency was the subject of the first clinical trial of gene therapy in 1990. Unfortunately, despite several subsequent trials, there is no convincing evidence that it has effected a cure, simply because there are too few cells in the circulation expressing the ADA gene. The problem, however, lies not with the concept but – like so much of biomedical research – with the application.

Requirements for successful gene therapy

For gene therapy to be successful, a thorough understanding of basic science issues is necessary:

- What is the nature of the disease?
- Is it genetic or acquired?
- Is it metabolic, structural or developmental? The first class will be relatively easy to treat, but the obstacles which must be overcome are by no means trivial. The second and third classes pose potentially insurmountable problems due to the irreversibility of many developmental defects and the need for precise regulation of gene expression (see Ref 4).
- How is the gene inherited?
- Is it dominant or recessive? The simple observation that one dose of a mutated gene is sufficient to cause a dominant disorder, whereas one copy of a normal gene is sufficient to mask a recessive trait, demonstrates immediately that these two situations pose fundamentally different obstacles with respect to gene dosage for phenotypic correction.
- What is the target tissue?
- Is the condition focal or systemic?
- Is one or more cell lineage affected?
- Is the gene product intracellular, extracellular or secreted?
- How will the gene be delivered? By aerosol, instillation, injection or orally? Or is surgery required to transplant or implant tissue that has been treated *ex vivo*?
- What vector will be used to deliver the gene?
- Will it be viral, perhaps a modified adenovirus, retrovirus or lentivirus, or a physical vectoring system such as cationic liposomes?
- What are the safety issues associated with each type of vector?
- Is there a window of opportunity between efficacy and toxicity that can be exploited?

All these questions have an important bearing upon the practicalities of developing a particular gene therapy strategy. The choice of vector will be determined by all the previous factors, plus the fundamental questions whether expression need only be transient or must be stable over the lifetime of the individual and whether the treatment can be administered just once or needs to be regularly repeated.

Definition of the gene

This general discussion takes us into the complicated area of what
defines the gene. The standard procedure is to link up a complementary DNA (cDNA) version of the messenger RNA (mRNA) to
suitable promoter and enhancer elements which will drive expression in the appropriate cell environment. The regulation of gene
expression is, however, much more complex. Promoter and
enhancer elements, which are important in physiological regulation, are immediately upstream and downstream of the coding
sequence. Other elements may be buried within the spacer DNA of
introns or lie far outside the obvious structural domain – the so-
called locus control regions. There is also growing evidence that
the local chromatin configuration and context are important in
gene regulation.

Thus, for practical purposes, it is necessary to start with simple
expression constructs, but to achieve sustained physiological levels
of expression it is likely that the endogenous gene will need to be
mimicked more closely. The first gene therapy company in the UK,
Therexsys, was launched on the back of key patents relating to
locus control regions.[5] They and many other laboratories are
putting significant effort into the manipulation for gene therapy of
genomic DNA fragments which retain all relevant regulatory
elements. These refinements lie in the future, however; for the
present, useful progress can be made with the viral and non-viral
reagents to hand.

Clinical targets for gene therapy

What gene therapy can and cannot do

What will be the first targets for treatment by gene therapy? It is
perhaps useful to start by saying what gene therapy can and cannot
do. Gene therapy can be used to:

- supply a missing gene,
- correct a biochemical, metabolic or physiological defect,
- add new gene products,
- improve natural defences, and/or
- kill cancer cells.

Gene therapy cannot be expected to repair damaged tissue or
reverse developmental birth defects.

The list of potential disease candidates for gene therapy is long,
and starts with the many single gene disorders considered

amenable to this form of intervention. It is noteworthy, however, that much of the research and most of the clinical trials so far have focused on the use of gene therapy as a new attack on cancer and viral infection.[6]

Cancer gene therapy

Antisense technology

Many strategies have been designed and are under test for cancer gene therapy. These include antisense technology in which an oligonucleotide complement to mRNA is synthesised and introduced into the target cell. The antisense oligonucleotide interacts in a highly specific fashion to block post-transcriptional processing or translation, specifically of the mutant but not of the wild type transcript.

Incidentally, there may be a role for antisense technology in the treatment of dominant disorders specifically to suppress transduction of mRNA transfer in the mutant allele.[1] Adding a missing tumour suppressor gene or additional counterbalancing copies of wild type proto-oncogenes may work in certain circumstances.

Anticancer gene therapy strategies

With cancer, though, there is an extreme version of the perennial problem of how to ensure gene delivery to a sufficient proportion of cells for clinical benefit. Consequently, most anticancer gene therapy strategies take a different approach to that of antisense technology. One solution is to target the gene therapy through receptors expressed specifically on cancer cells. The gene is not therapeutic in the normal sense, but is a 'suicide' gene which may have a direct killing effect or activate an otherwise harmless pro-drug. In this way, only the proliferating cancer cells are killed and normal tissue is spared.

It might be questioned whether this strategy could ever be sufficiently efficient to target all tumour cells. A surprising, but beneficial observation is the so-called 'bystander' effect: for each cancer cell targeted and killed, many more surrounding cancer cells also die by a mechanism which is poorly understood but is probably, at least in part, immunological. This strategy may have a valuable role to play in treating inoperable solid tumours, but it does not address the major issue of metastatic spread. The immune system can also be used directly to fight the cancer, and may be more appropriate in this regard. The tumour cells are made to express an antigen which primes the immune system to recognise not just the transfected cancer cell but also the remaining bulk of tumour mass and, potentially, secondary metastases.

As an adjunct to conventional therapy

A different general anticancer strategy is to use gene therapy as an adjunct to conventional therapy, with the aim of protecting the normal proliferating cells, notably haemopoietic cell lineages, from the toxic effects of chemotherapy or radiation therapy. This is an attractive approach because it can be seen as a logical addition to, rather than unproven substitute for, well established clinical practice.

The role of animal models in developing gene therapy: the cystic fibrosis paradigm*

Developing cancer gene therapy highlights a significant problem facing the development of any new form of treatment: how to translate into clinical practice good ideas and experimental evidence gleaned from the laboratory. Animal studies are an important intermediate. In this regard, the cancer field in general, and the gene therapy field in particular, need better animal models. These may come as a spin-off from the Human Genome Project because of the importance attached to the comparative study of other species. For example, genetic engineering can be used to create mouse models of genetic conditions more or less at will.[7]

Animal models of cystic fibrosis (CF) illustrate several key points in relation to gene therapy.[8] These models have been created by gene targeting in embryonic stem cells. A fragment of the murine CF gene is introduced into cultured embryonal stem cells. Individual clones are selected which have taken up the DNA and incorporated it specifically into the endogenous mouse CF gene. The process of integration by genetic recombination disrupts the gene, so these cells are effectively now 'carriers' of the CF mutation. The cells can be recovered as viable, pure-breeding animals in two generations of breeding:

---

*See Chapter 4 for more general discussion of cystic fibrosis

1   Chimeras are formed by injection of the gene targeted cells into host blastocysts.
2   The chimeric mice are backcrossed to appropriate breeder stocks.

If the gene targeted embryonal stem cells contribute to the germline, pure breeding 'carrier' mice are produced which, on intercrossing, segregate in a 1:2:1 fashion for CF homozygote, heterozygote and wild type mice. The same scheme can be applied to the targeted disruption of any chosen gene.

The CF mutant mice display many of the key features of the disease exhibited in patients, including the electrophysiological defect in the respiratory and intestinal tracts, perinatal intestinal disease, reduced respiratory mucociliary clearance, and susceptibility to lung infection with CF-associated pathogens.[9] Gene targeting can be used to introduce mutations in a way which does not completely obliterate gene function but rather modulates it in both quality and quantity.[10,11]

The next question is how the modulation of CF gene activity relates to the phenotype, either measured close to the gene in terms of electrophysiological ion channel activity or more distally in terms of intestinal disease. The observed relationships are distinctly non-linear. The non-linearity is more striking with more (phenotypic) steps removed from the primary defect.[12] Thus, whereas with 5% of normal levels of CF gene activity there is only partial correction of the electrophysiological defect, the intestinal disease is completely corrected. This is encouraging because it argues that just a few per cent correction by somatic gene therapy would have a substantial clinical impact.

This conclusion is in keeping with other clinical and experimental evidence,[13,14] but begs the question of whether all cells must express at least 5% of normal levels or whether 5% of all cells expressing high levels of the CF gene would have an equivalent effect. Our inability, as yet, to answer this question satisfactorily reflects a lack of certainty (true for many single gene and multifactorial disorders) about the relative contribution of gene expression in different cell types to the physiological manifestation of the disease. This is one obvious and important question to be addressed by the 'post-genome' challenge through functional genetics.

From basic science to clinical application

Cationic liposomes

Most investigators in the USA concentrated initially on using

recombinant adenovirus to deliver the CF gene (see Re
for review). The UK focus has been on cationic liposor
the advantages of this approach being ease of manufactur ﹍
use, chemical definition and flexibility of design. Cationic liposomes also avoid the twin problems of an immunological and host
response to adenoviral infection which blunts the biological
response and exacerbates the inflammatory response. The down-
side is their relative inefficiency. Nevertheless, aerosolised delivery
of reporter genes to'the mouse gave encouraging gene delivery
and expression.[16] When the CF gene itself was used, correction of
the electrophysiological defect in CF mutant mice was observed.[17,18]

These results led to the first Phase 1 study of gene therapy in the
UK involving a single dose of DNA/liposome applied to the nose
of CF patients,[19] closely followed by similar studies at additional UK
centres.[20,21] All three studies produced comparable results. There
was little, if any, evidence for inflammatory response attributable to
treatment. Although the evidence for gene transfer and expression
was encouraging, the responses were incomplete and transient.
Nevertheless, they were at least as good as any of the adenoviral
studies, and sufficiently encouraging to justify studies of cationic
liposome-mediated gene delivery to the CF lung. Alton and
colleagues at the Royal Brompton Hospital have just completed a
single-dose study to the lung in collaboration with Genzyme
Corporation, while the Edinburgh group is in the advanced
planning stages of a dose escalation study of gene delivery to the
lung.

Development of a clinically available gene therapy for cystic fibrosis

Useful progress has thus been made in the first stage of developing
CF gene therapy as a new form of treatment for this life-shortening
condition. It is important to emphasise the logistical difficulties of
progressing from this stage all the way through to the development
of a drug which can be used reliably and effectively. Many scientific
barriers have yet to be overcome before we can be confident that
we have a product that can be administered safely and repeatedly,
that can penetrate the protective (and infected) barrier of the
epithelial lining fluid, target the appropriate secretory epithelial
cells, cross the cell membrane, escape the endosome, traverse the
cytoplasm, pass through the nuclear membrane and express stably
and undamaged in the nucleus.

This will be an iterative process involving much more basic
laboratory science and incorporating findings from the various

ongoing Phase 1 and Phase 2 studies here and abroad. Significant improvements will no doubt be required in each component and in formulating the chosen combination of gene and vector. Industrial 'know how' is vital because, in terms of quality assurance and formulation, gene therapy development has many similarities to conventional drug development. In the long term, collaboration between basic and clinical scientists and between academia and industry will be required for success.[22]

The need for improved animal models and gene therapy strategies

There will be a continuing need for relevant animal studies, as far as possible using genetic models. For the moment, this restricts us almost entirely to the laboratory mouse because efficient embryonal stem cell gene targeting and saturation chemical mutagenesis is possible only in this species. In an ideal world, however, it would often be preferable to use a species whose size and physiology matched more closely that of humans. The sheep would be close to an ideal model for CF. The technology which gave rise to Dolly,[23] and sparked such controversy by raising the spectre of human cloning and designer babies, may in fact hold the key to a better understanding of many fundamental biological processes.[24] In the present context, it does not take a leap of imagination to propose genetic modification of cultured sheep cells to create precise mutations, using the nuclear transplantation technology to derive a mutant sheep.

Finally, and for the future, perhaps the technology used to generate transgenic animal models might be applied in reverse for precise gene therapy. In essence, this would involve identifying and isolating somatic stem cells from affected tissues, propagating these in the laboratory and using gene targeting, not to introduce but to correct the mutation precisely. The loop would be closed, and a genuine cure at the organ level effected by engraftment of the corrected somatic stem cells. Although futuristic, valuable progress is being made towards these ends using, as always, the laboratory mouse to research and develop these revolutionary ideas.[25]

Conclusions

In conclusion, gene therapy still has some way to go before it will be part of standard clinical practice, but a wealth of enthusiasm and bright ideas are making steady progress towards that aim. It is not a 'cure all', but rather one more significant addition to the armoury which is highly relevant to a significant subset of genetic and acquired diseases. Individuals and families affected by genetic diseases look to the clinical and scientific community for hope. Striking the right balance between optimism and realism is difficult, but necessary. Progress will not be made without the selfless cooperation of affected individuals. Many genetic conditions, individually rare but collectively large (comprising one in 100 of the population), will never be considered commercially viable in terms of conventional drug development. The hope is that, with gene therapy at least, generic approaches will be developed which can be effectively and economically adapted for these rare conditions.

To put all this into practice, however, will depend heavily upon a welfare health service such as the UK NHS. When the genome science has matured and gene therapy has been perfected, it is vital that the NHS remains intact and able to put all this good research into ethical and equitable practice.

References

1 Porteous DJ. From genes to therapy. *The Biochemist* 1993; October/November: 16–9.
2 Verma IM. Gene therapy. *Scientific American* 1990; November: 34–41.
3 Crystal RG. Transfer of genes to humans: early lessons and obstacles to success. *Science* 1995; **270**: 404–10.
4 Millington-Ward S, O'Neill B, Tuohy G, Al-Jandal N, *et al*. Stratagems in vitro for gene therapies directed to dominant mutations. *Human Molecular Genetics* 1997; **6**: 1415–26.
5 *MRC News* 1993; **60**: 27. (Free copies from: The Publications Group, Medical Research Council, 20 Park Crescent, London W1N 4AL.)
6 *MRC News* 1994; **62**: (entire Spring issue).
7 Brandon EP, Idzerda RL, Mcknight GS. Targeting the mouse genome – a compendium of knockouts. *Current Biology* 1995; **5**: 1073.
8 McLachlan G, Porteous DJ, Houdebine LM (eds). The role of mouse models in the development of new therapies for cystic fibrosis. In: *Transgenic animals: generation and use*. Amsterdam: Harwood Academic Press, 1997: 435–44.
9 Davidson DJ, Dorin JR, McLachlan G, Ranaldi V, *et al*. Lung disease in the cystic fibrosis mouse exposed to bacterial pathogens. *Nature Genetics* 1995; **9**: 351–7.
10 Dorin JR, Dickinson P, Alton EWFW, Smith SN, *et al*. Cystic fibrosis in the mouse by targeted insertional mutagenesis. *Nature* 1992; **359**: 211–5.
11 Delaney SJ, Alton EWFW, Smith SN, *et al*. Cystic-fibrosis mice carrying the missense mutation G551D replicate human genotype-phenotype correlations. *EMBO Journal* 1996; **15**: 955–63.
12 Dorin JR, Farley R, Webb S, Smith SN, *et al*. A demonstration using mouse models that successful gene therapy for cystic fibrosis requires only partial gene correction. *Gene Therapy* 1996; **3**: 797–801.

13 Chu C-S, Trapnell BC, Curristin S, Cutting GR, Crystal RG. Genetic basis of variable exon 9 skipping in cystic fibrosis transmembrane conductance regulator mRNA. *Nature Genetics* 1993; **3**: 151–6.

14 Johnson LG, Olsen JC, Sarkadi B, Moore KL, *et al.* Efficiency of gene-transfer for restoration of normal airway epithelial function in cystic fibrosis. *Nature Genetics* 1992; **2**: 21–5.

15 Wilson JM. Gene therapy for cystic fibrosis: challenges and future directions. *Journal of Clinical Investigation* 1995; **96**: 2547–54.

16 McLachlan G, Davidson DJ, Stevenson BJ, Dickinson P, *et al.* Evaluation *in vitro* and *in vivo* of cationic liposome-expression construct complexes for cystic fibrosis gene therapy. *Gene Therapy* 1995; **2**: 614–22.

17 Hyde SC, Gill DR, Higgins CF, Trezise AEO, *et al.* Correction of the ion-transport defect in cystic-fibrosis transgenic mice by gene-therapy. *Nature* 1993; **362**: 250–5.

18 Govan JRW, Brown PH, Maddison J, Doherty CJ, *et al.* Evidence for transmission of Pseudomonas-cepacia by social contact in cystic fibrosis. *Lancet* 1993; **342**: 15–9.

19 Caplen NJ, Alton EWFW, Middleton PG, Dorin JR, *et al.* Liposome-mediated *CFTR* gene transfer to the nasal epithelium of patients with cystic fibrosis. *Nature Medicine* 1995; **1**: 39–46.

20 Gill DR, Southern KW, Mofford KA, Seddon T, *et al.* A placebo controlled study of liposome-mediated gene transfer to the nasal epithelium of patients with cystic fibrosis. *Gene Therapy* 1997; **4**: 199–209.

21 Porteous DJ, Dorin JR, McLachlan G, Davidson-Smith H, *et al.* Evidence for the safety and efficacy of DOTAP cationic liposome mediated *CFTR* gene transfer to the nasal epithelium of patients with cystic fibrosis. *Gene Therapy* 1997; **4**: 210–8.

22 Rigby PWJ. Gene therapy: a long and winding road. *Current Opinion in Genetics and Development* 1995; **5**: 397–8.

23 Wilmut I, Schnieke AE, McWhir J, Kind AJ, Campbell KHS. Viable offspring derived from fetal and adult mammalian cells. *Nature* 1997; **385**: 810–3.

24 Butler D, Wadman M. Putting the lid on Pandora's box of genetics. *Nature* 1997; **386**: 9.

25 Slorach EM, Dorin JR, Halter F, Winton D, Wright NA (eds). Towards gene correction for cystic fibrosis in intestinal stem cells. In: *The gut as a model in cell and molecular biology*, 1st edn. Hingham, USA: Kluwer Academic Publishers, 1997: 34–46.

19 | The public understanding of genetics*

Tom Wilkie
Biomedical Ethics Section, The Wellcome Trust, London

The principal theme of this chapter is ignorance. Despite its commitment to empirical evidence gathering, the scientific community has been surprisingly unscientific in its approach to the public understanding of science. Scientists in receipt of funds from the public purse have tended to lag behind industry as well as central and local government in the study of public attitudes and opinion. Industrial and commercial companies must confront the reality of public opinion directly; they depend upon consumers buying their products. In contrast, bench scientists are, rightly, shielded by institutions such as the research councils from having to pursue topics which may transiently have caught the popular imagination, but this can sometimes shade, wrongly, into isolation from the concerns of the scientists' ultimate paymasters, the public.[1]

Early attempts

The deficit model

Public understanding of science as an academic discipline is really only just over 10 years old. It started with the Bodmer Report to the Royal Society in 1985.[2] For the first few years, however, it set off down something of a blind alley, perhaps understandably concentrating on what is now called the 'deficit model' of public understanding. This view holds that the public is deficient in factual knowledge on scientific topics, that this deficiency can be measured, and all that is required to enhance the public understanding of science is to 'educate' the public to see scientific topics in the way that the scientists themselves see them.

---

*The views reported in this chapter are solely those of the author, and do not reflect the policies or outlook of the Wellcome Trust.

The apogee of this theory was represented in the survey conducted in 1988 as part of the British Social Attitudes survey.[3,4] This asked a series of factual questions, including ones designed to elucidate whether respondents understood that the earth went round the sun once a year. There was consternation when less than a third of the population answered correctly. Following that, a survey[5] was conducted in Scotland for the Edinburgh science festival which discovered that few Scots could name a living scientist. Many thought that Albert Einstein, who died in 1955, was still alive and well.

A failure to disaggregate 'the public'

A second false start, from which we still suffer today, was a failure to disaggregate the public. Society does not consist of a priest-hood of the scientifically literate, outside whose temples (research laboratories) there is some lumpenproletariat sunk in ignorance and superstition. In fact, people congregate together into interest groups and lobby groups, and they also differentiate according to age, social class and gender. The interests and attitudes of a 20 year old single male are rather different from those of a 45 year old married male with two young children even if they both live in London. For example, there is a clear age gap in expectations of medical research: cancer is the highest priority of younger groups who do not mention cardiovascular conditions at all, whereas older age groups have a preoccupation with medical research for heart disease (Wellcome Trust research; to be published in 1998). These interests and attitudes affect risk-taking behaviour and expectations of what the health service, food manufacturers and other institutions of society might deliver.

The media and education of the public

These two failings, concentration on the deficit model and a fail-ure to disaggregate the public, led to ultimately futile interventions to influence and 'educate' them. Attempts were made to reach the public directly through exhibitions and events on the street. How-ever, distribution systems already exist for spreading information to the broad mass of the public at large – that is, via newspapers, radio and television.[6]

Two features about the media make them inappropriate vehicles for getting over the sort of message considered necessary within the deficit model of public understanding of science: first, the media rightly guard their editorial control. Thus, scientists who expect to get a pedagogic message directly across to the mass of the public framed from their own perspective find instead that it is filtered, criticised and commented upon.

Secondly, with regard to the disaggregation of the public, even among the mass media there is no one public. The readership of the *Daily Telegraph*, for example, is different and distinct from that of *The Guardian*. Editors of newspapers are acutely aware of this dis-aggregation, and choose the stories which they will run accordingly. For example, the *Daily Telegraph* has reported HIV/AIDS sparsely compared to the attention given to this issue by *The Guardian* and *The Independent*. In fact, the HIV/AIDS story well illustrates the way in which editors choose the story and its treatment – the way in which some event is reported and commented upon, and the prominence given to it – in accordance with their view of the interests of their readers. In contrast, in the early days of the public understanding of science programme, there was little recognition of this necessity to tailor a message to 'consumer demand'.

Gradually, however, the realisation dawned that researchers were asking the wrong questions. Various segments of the public did have an understanding of science, but a subtle and complex one. More particularly, the public brought to an assessment of scientific and technological issues criteria which were different to those the scientists would have deemed appropriate or relevant. For many of the public, these different perspectives may be more important than the scientists' perspective. The filtration, criticism and commentary necessary to purvey messages through the mass media reflect the media's view of their readers' agendas. The media will thus present scientific news and information from the perspective of the reader, not from that of the scientist.

Risk assessment and perception

The importance of non-scientific issues is well illustrated by the general example of risk assessment and perception. Society accepts different sorts of risks for reasons of historical accident, economic structure and perception of benefit. Thus, smoking has not been banned because of the weight of economic and historical background. British Nuclear Fuels' reprocessing plant at Sellafield in West Cumbria, on the other hand, represents comparatively little risk but has garnered a great deal of unpopularity, among the reasons for which must surely be included historical perceptions of the link between civilian nuclear power and nuclear weapons, and the inability of people to exercise consumer choice. Consumers can buy petrol at a station other than Esso out of protest at the Exxon Valdez oil spill, but they cannot exclude every fourth electron from the socket in their wall.

The general point is that the 'scientific' perception that a calculus of comparative risks is all that matters (eg see Ref 7) is not congruent with that of the public. Furthermore, the public's perception is not necessarily either arbitrary or illogical.

The abandonment of the deficit model opened the way to understanding some results which would otherwise appear inconsistent and paradoxical, one of the most striking of which is that some sectors of the public actively maintain ignorance of some scientific issues. The best example comes from a study conducted by Wynne among apprentices at the Sellafield reprocessing plant.[8] He found that they actively did not want to know the relationship between radiation and cancer. The knowledge would have been too disturbing for them to have continued working there. Relevant knowledge for the apprentices was an assurance that their employer had procedures in place to protect their health, and that these were monitored and vetted by the Nuclear Installations Inspectorate and other regulatory bodies. What was relevant to them was 'social' rather than technical knowledge: information and understanding about the mechanisms of control which society had put in place, so that they could have confidence in the institutional control of their risks.

Increasing public concern accompanies increasing knowledge

A second apparently paradoxical result is that increasing knowledge does not correlate with increasing acceptance of science and technology. On the contrary, a consistent finding of several studies is that it is associated with increasing concern, amounting in some cases to opposition to science and science-based industry. Examples, drawn again from the nuclear industry, are evident from the research by Lee from the University of St Andrews.[9,10] Lee and his colleagues found that a UK Atomic Energy Authority (UKAEA) stand at the Ideal Home Exhibition attracted people concerned about nuclear power, who became more concerned after visiting the exhibition than they had been before (TD Lee, D Uzzell; unpublished report to the UKAEA, 1985).

Both these results are inexplicable within the context of the 'deficit model.' Once that model is abandoned, however, they make sense and show that public responses to scientific and technical information are often well informed and intelligent. The framework and perspective applied, however, may differ from the scientist's and may attach far higher importance to non-technical information. Thus, the public response to any new scientific information is likely to be much richer and more complex than might be expected on the basis of the deficit model.

The purpose of this long but necessary preamble has been to suggest that any statements about what are the 'public expectations' or 'public understanding' of genetics must be tentative. A significant compendium of the research which has been done is contained in *The troubled helix*,[11] a book which represents an essential starting point in this field.

The rest of this chapter will first discuss three recent and sophisticated efforts to gauge the public mood in relation to genetics and its applications:

1. A paper by Richards in *Public Understanding of Science* in 1996.[12]
2. A paper on public attitudes in *Nature* in 1997.[13]
3. 'The people decide', a deliberative poll organised by the Wellcome Trust, also in 1997.[14]

The chapter will conclude by describing the efforts now under way inside the Wellcome Trust to try to achieve a more sophisticated understanding of the public and of its expectations.

Lay knowledge of genetics

Richards[12] sought to explain and make sense of the limited understanding of Mendelian genetics that he and other researchers had found among schoolchildren, adults and those offered genetic counselling. He reported preliminary empirical work among various 'publics':

- 30 women coming to a family history clinic for breast cancer counselling;
- 30 families suffering from neurofibromatosis;
- 200 members of the Women's Institute; and
- 80 first-year social science undergraduates.

As an example of the results, only 29% of those attending a Women's Institute conference on the new genetics understood that an individual shares 50% of his/her genes with siblings, but 90% got the father/child relationship correct. Given that these women were attending a conference on genetics, they might be expected already to have a particular interest in the subject and perhaps to perform better than the 'non-attentive' public. This hypothesis was indeed borne out by the observation that only 9% of the friends of those attending the conference gave a correct answer about siblings.

Richards put forward the view that Mendelian explanations of inheritance conflict in several respects with a lay knowledge of inheritance widespread in society. Moreover, the lay ideas about inheritance are grounded in concepts of kinship which reflect everyday social practice in society. It is no mere accident that the English language uses the same word, 'inheritance', for the transmission of biological characteristics across generations and for the passing on of goods and chattels to one's heirs.

It is for this reason that the lay perception places the genetic connection between parents and offspring closer than the genetic connection between siblings. If this empirical work is correct, it means that much of the theory of 'sociobiology' is wrong. Sociobiology suggests that much of human social behaviour follows from genetic and evolutionary causes, and that many social relationships are merely manifestations of genes maximising their survival. Richards' work, however, suggests that kin relationships in our society are not determined by the genetic link. Rather, it is the other way round: people's understanding of their genetic links is conditioned by the closeness of their kinship ties.

A second point is that humans are not like pea plants: very few human characteristics are transmitted in a straightforward Mendelian single-gene fashion. The common experience is of characteristics such as height which are under polygenic (and environmental) control. In the lay experience, without mathematical demonstration, the Mendelian picture does not obviously apply to humans.

The suggestion that perceived biological relatedness derives from the strength of social connections makes sense of many problems in the public understanding of genetics which are otherwise difficult to explain. It accounts for the failure of formal education over the past several decades to instil basic Mendelian concepts, and for the persistent problems in getting over concepts of risk during genetic counselling sessions. For example, the concept of recessive characteristics is not generally appreciated, a specific example being the very real possibility that daughters of fathers who are carriers of the BRCA mutation may not be warned that they are at risk.

Part of the difficulty may be that current analogies are misleading. Terms such as 'plan' and 'blueprint' reinforce erroneous genetic determinism. Richards suggests that a better way of conveying genetic information is to build on and extend existing lay knowledge, facing head on the problem of segregating characters (such as eye colour) and those which appear to mix and blend (such as facial appearance and body build). Whether highly technical genetic information is needed at all in the course of genetic counselling sessions is, in his view, very much a live issue.

Public attitudes

The 3rd Eurobarometer survey

Reference has been made several times to the possible disconnection between technical knowledge and positive or negative public attitudes towards genetics, but precisely what *are* public attitudes? Some information was produced as a result of the 3rd Eurobarometer survey, conducted in October/November 1996;[13] the two earlier surveys were conducted in 1991 and 1993.

A random sample of 16,246 people across Europe aged 15 years or above (ca 1,000 from each European Union member state) was taken, and the individuals questioned about their attitudes to various aspects of genetics and biotechnology. Technical knowledge was not the prime focus of this research.

Biotechnology was divided into the three main areas of medical applications, agriculture/food and animal research (taken to include xenotransplantation). Respondents were asked to describe their view of these aspects of biotechnology as useful, risky, morally acceptable, or to be encouraged.

In the area of medical applications, there was a large positive support for genetic testing and genetically-based medicines, and the medical profession was widely trusted. However, with regard to agriculture and food, the European public were ambivalent about crop and food production, and it was the environmental groups who were trusted here. Animal experiments were regarded as risky, immoral and to be discouraged – this applied both to the use of animals in research and xenografts. Perhaps a little paradoxically, animal welfare groups and universities were both trusted.

On the trustworthiness index, there were some possibly surprising results. Although, as customary in such surveys, journalists were held in low esteem, TV and newspapers scored more highly than industry, religion or politicians. The highest trustworthiness scores were for environmental and consumer groups, followed by the medical profession.

Attitudes to regulation were interesting. Perhaps in recognition that science is international, the idea of transboundary regulation was popular. The ranking order for regulation is shown in Table 1.

One primary consideration was the need for public control. There were strongly supported sentiments in favour of labelling on genetically modified food (74%), public consultation on biotechnology (60%), and on the insufficiency of current regulations (53%).

The researchers' primary conclusion, however, was that risk is not the crucial factor. Instead, they believe their results show that 'moral doubts act as a veto irrespective of people's views on usefulness and risk'. They suggest that, because biotechnology regulation focuses on risk – a technical matter – and not on morality, much of the current thrust of European regulation is misplaced.

Gauging the public mood

In recent years, considerable interest has been shown by many areas of society in developing methods of sounding out public opinion directly. Several innovative methodologies have been tried, such as citizens' juries, deliberative polls and focus group discussions. It is worth noting that some of this may at least imply that the traditional, constitutional methods of representing public views and public opinions, by the election of members of parliament and local councillors, are failing to deliver. A more positive view might be that these developments reflect an increasing democratisation of society as people take more interest in the decisions made in their name.

Table 1. Attitudes to regulation among the general public in the European Union countries.[13]

Order of ranking	Organisation	%
1	International bodies	35
2	Scientific organisations	25
3	National public bodies	12
4	Ethics committees	10
5	European Union	9
6	National parliaments	6

Common to many of these approaches is the belief that simple opinion poll survey methods are inadequate to deal with novel or complex issues. By their very nature, quantitative opinion polls condition and restrict the possible responses. There is no scope for the respondent to say 'yes, but ...'. When issues as new as modern genetics and their social implications are on the agenda, there is a need for people to discuss, check technical points and hear the opinions of others before they can be sure of their own minds. None of these things is possible in quantitative opinion polls and, although the numbers may be statistically significant, their results need to be interpreted with care.

In March 1997, the Wellcome Trust embarked on an exercise to probe the ideas and values behind the overt responses.[14] During National Science Week, it organised a deliberative poll, and assembled approximately 400 people in Westminster Hall, London. The sample was selected to be as representative as possible of the population of London (although, inevitably, those who actually make the effort to come will not be fully representative). First, the audience heard from expert witnesses, and then discussed the issues amongst themselves. Finally, a series of questions were put to them, upon which they voted using a hand-held electronic device which allowed instantaneous display of the result. There was thus deliberation as well as polling.

The results included:

- an agreement that there should be no genetic discrimination in insurance;
- a division of opinion about the cloning of Dolly and on whether research is going too far; and
- opposition to research into the genetic basis of intelligence and depression.

This deliberative poll was conducted shortly after the cloning of Dolly had hit the headlines, and the division among the audience about whether or not this had been a good development was in marked contrast to the press coverage which had been critical of it.

Advances during the past decade

Over the past decade, research work on the public understanding of science has gradually begun to show that the public response to science and technology is richer and more complex than was assumed at the time of the Bodmer report.[2] Some publics are simply inattentive, whereas others actively maintain ignorance of scientific matters. Those publics which do engage with science and technology bring their own values and perspectives to the debate, and ultimately will not accept that debate being confined to aspects deemed relevant by the scientific community. Science itself is ill-served if scientists ignore or try to divert discussion from the issues considered relevant by the public.

One of the most interesting findings is that *technical* issues of risk assessment are not really relevant in public attitudes to any technology, and specifically to genetics. Risk has two components:

- the 'technical' assessment of the probability of an event taking place, and
- the severity or unacceptability of the event itself.

Two events may have widely differing probabilities of occurring but, if the less probable is considered unacceptable, public judgement will focus on the event and not on its probability. This is not an irrational or innumerate response, but an expression of choice. The mathematical calculus of probability is less important than the moral calculus of ethical values.

The other fundamental discovery of the past decade has been that public attitudes do not correlate well with degree of technical knowledge. There is thus a need to address directly the public's attitudes to science and technology, as distinct from measuring technical competence in understanding the scientific details.

Future developments

The Wellcome Trust is developing a programme in the social and ethical consequences of biomedical advance. It will be complemented by social research into public attitudes and the values, feelings and cultural influences which form those judgements on science and technology. In this way, a 'practical' ethics will be developed in which public understanding is taken to encompass not just the technical but the moral understanding of genetics.

References

1 Shils E. The public understanding of science. *Minerva* 1974; **12**: 153–8.
2 Bodmer W (Chairman). *The public understanding of science.* Report of a Royal Society *ad hoc* group, endorsed by the Council of the Royal Society. London: Royal Society, 1985.
3 Evans G, Durant J. Understanding of science in Britain and the USA.

In: *British social attitudes. Special international report.* London: SCPR, Gower Publishing, 1989: Ch 6.

4   Durant J, Evans G, Thomas GP. The public understanding of science. *Nature* 1989; **340**: 11–4.

5   *Public awareness of science in Scotland.* Research results, Scotinform Ltd, 1991.

6   *Communicating science to the public.* Ciba Foundation Conference. New York: John Wiley, 1987.

7   Health and Safety Executive. *Tolerability of risk from nuclear power stations.* London: HMSO, 1988.

8   Wynne B. Public understanding of science research: new horizons or hall of mirrors? *Public understanding of science.* 1992; **1**: 37–43.

9   Lee T, Balchin N. Learning and attitude change at British Nuclear Fuels Sellafield Visitors' Centre. *Journal of Environmental Psychology* 1995; **15**: 283–98.

10 Lee T. Communications breakdown in nuclear energy. *Physics World* No. 2, April 1989: 25–6.

11 Marteau T, Richards M (eds). *The troubled helix: social and psychological implications of the new human genetics.* Cambridge: Cambridge University Press, 1996.

12 Richards M. Lay and professional knowledge of genetics and inheritance. *Public Understanding of Science* 1996; **5**: 217–30.

13 Biotechnology and the European Public Concerted Action Group. Europe ambivalent on biotechnology. *Nature* 1997; **387**: 845–7.

14 *The people decide.* Report on the event. London: Wellcome Trust, 19 March 1997.

Appendix

Tools of the trade

Chris Mathew and Andrew Read

The basic questions which the clinician needs to be able to answer to derive the maximum benefit from this book can be stated as follows:

- What is the structure of a gene?
- How is a gene expressed?
- What kind of structural alterations (mutations) may occur in a gene to affect its function?
- What are DNA polymorphisms, and how can they be used to locate disease genes?
- How are disease genes cloned?
- How are the variations of DNA sequence (mutations or polymorphisms) detected in the laboratory?

The answers to these questions can be found in a wide variety of reviews and textbooks, some of which are listed below. The choice will depend upon the enthusiasm and the budget of the reader.

Introductory reviews in journals and books

Savill J. Science, medicine and the future. *British Medical Journal* 1997; **314**:
- pages 43–5. Prospecting for gold in the human genome.
- pages 126–9. Molecular genetic approaches to understanding disease.
- pages 203–6. Role of molecular cell biology in understanding disease.

Read AP. Molecular genetics and inherited human diseasae. In: Thakker RV (ed). *Molecular genetics of endocrine disorders*. London: Chapman & Hall, 1997.

Introductory textbooks

Brock DJH. *Molecular genetics for the clinician*. Cambridge: Cambridge University Press, 1993.
Emery A, Malcolm S. *An introduction to recombinant DNA*, 2nd edn. Chichester: John Wiley, 1995.

Muller RF, Young ID. *Emery's elements of medical genetics*, 10th edn. Edinburgh: Churchill Livingstone, 1998.

Comprehensive textbook

Strachan T, Read AP. *Human molecular genetics*. Oxford: Bios Scientific Publishers Ltd, 1996.